Abortion Trail Activism

Abortion Trail Activism

*The Global Infrastructures
for Abortion Access*

Deirdre Niamh Duffy

BLOOMSBURY ACADEMIC
LONDON • NEW YORK • OXFORD • NEW DELHI • SYDNEY

BLOOMSBURY ACADEMIC
Bloomsbury Publishing Plc
50 Bedford Square, London, WC1B 3DP, UK
1385 Broadway, New York, NY 10018, USA
29 Earlsfort Terrace, Dublin 2, Ireland

BLOOMSBURY, BLOOMSBURY ACADEMIC and the Diana logo are trademarks of Bloomsbury Publishing Plc

First published in Great Britain 2024

Copyright © Deirdre Niamh Duffy, 2024

Deirdre Niamh Duffy has asserted her right under the Copyright, Designs and Patents Act, 1988, to be identified as Author of this work.

For legal purposes the Acknowledgements on p. xi constitute an extension of this copyright page.

Cover design by Adriana Brioso
Cover image © Dedraw Studio/Adobe Stock

Bloomsbury Publishing Plc does not have any control over, or responsibility for, any third-party websites referred to or in this book. All internet addresses given in this book were correct at the time of going to press. The author and publisher regret any inconvenience caused if addresses have changed or sites have ceased to exist, but can accept no responsibility for any such changes.

This work is published open access subject to a Creative Commons Attribution 4.0 licence (CC BY 4.0, https://creativecommons.org/licenses/by/4.0/). You may re-use, distribute, reproduce, and adapt this work in any medium, including for commercial purposes, provided you give attribution to the copyright holder and the publisher, provide a link to the Creative Commons licence, and indicate if changes have been made.

A catalogue record for this book is available from the British Library.

Library of Congress Cataloging-in-Publication Data

ISBN: HB: 978-1-3502-4700-0
PB: 978-1-3502-4699-7
ePDF: 978-1-3502-4702-4
eBook: 978-1-3502-4701-7

Typeset by Deanta Global Publishing Services, Chennai, India
Printed and bound in Great Britain

To find out more about our authors and books visit www.bloomsbury.com and sign up for our newsletters.

Dedication

For Róisín, Fergus and Dónal – I hope you read this when you are older. I am sorry it is not a real storybook and that I do not mention Boudicca.

For Mark – Don't worry, I will not make you read it.

For abortion trail activists everywhere.

Author biography

Deirdre Niamh Duffy is a Senior Lecturer in Sociology at Lancaster University. She graduated with a PhD from University of Nottingham, an MSc Econ from Aberystwyth University, Aberystwyth, Wales, UK, and a BA (Hons) from University College Cork, Cork, Ireland. She is from Navan, the best town in Ireland.

She previously worked at Manchester Metropolitan University and Edge Hill University, Ormskirk, England. She collaborated on the first independent reviews of abortion services in the Republic of Ireland following the repeal of the Eighth Amendment.

She lives in a forest, enjoys picnics, hates the patriarchy and spends far too much time thinking about access to abortion.

Someone you love has had an abortion – *Abortion activist proverb*

Contents

Author biography	vi
Acknowledgements	xi
Introduction	1
Four accounts of abortion trail activism	1
Abortion trail activism	16
Structure of the book	28
Methodology, positionality and language-use statement	32
1 Access	37
Introduction	37
A shared activism	38
Understanding accessibility	43
Abortion trail activism and accessibility as a political intervention	59
Conclusion	64
2 Care	67
Introduction	67
On Aunties	68
Understanding a feminist, non-normative care ontology	77
Practising feminist care ethics	88
Conclusions	98
3 Prefiguring Abortion Infrastructures	101
Introduction	101
Understanding prefigurative politics	102
Reading abortion trail activism as prefigurative	109
Conclusions	120
4 Abortion trails and the Narrative of Pro-Choice	125
Introduction	125
Abortion trails and the narratives of pro-choice	126

Framings of abortion trails	131
Narrating pro-choice intents through abortion trails	146
5 Pro-choice Abortion Projects and The Problematic Politics of Tidying Abortion Trails	151
Introduction	151
Narrative, pro-choice abortion politics and abortion trails	153
Pro-choice abortion developments and the interpretation of abortion trails	158
What counts as a formal abortion architecture?	163
Limitations of a formal architecture	166
Conclusion: Why pursue formalization?	171
Conclusion	175
Why abortion trail activism?	179
Understanding abortion trail activism	180
The analytic value of abortion trail activism	181
Abortion trail activism and the pro-choice project	182
Bibliography	185
Index	206

Acknowledgements

Writing a book takes a village and there are dozens of people who have made this book possible.

My thanks go to my research participants, the relevant funding bodies (the Leverhulme Trust and the Wellcome Trust) and the institutions where I worked during this project. I would particularly like to thank Lancaster University for giving me the space to complete the manuscript and my colleagues in sociology for pushing me towards the end (special mentions to Michaela Benson and Aaron Winter for listening to me complain).

I obviously extend my huge appreciation to everyone who listened to my rambling thoughts, read drafts and provided feedback through the process. I can highly recommend Claire Pierson, Rishita Nandagiri, Natalie Hammond and Monique Huysamen as patient and supportive sounding boards.

I have been lucky enough to collaborate – and hopefully am lucky enough to continue these collaborations – as part of the projects that this book was fuelled by, with some phenomenal researchers, scholars and activists including Diana Lopez Castaneda, Megan Daigle, Ernestina Coast, Lucia Berro Pizzarossa and Judicaelle Irakoze.

Academics cannot exist on intellectual conversations alone and I am beyond thankful for the fantastic friends who have cheered me on throughout. Dr Sarah Pollock – I can never possibly repay you for listening to every single voice-note (including the ones that made no sense). Especially when they came in almost hourly towards the end. Thanks also to Máiread Enright, Fiona de Londras and Aoife O'Donoghue for your reassurance and your friendship and to Leanne O'Leary and Aine Clancy for your writing (and emotional) support.

And final thanks, as always, go to my family, who put up with my regular absence and occasional borderline neglect.

Introduction

Four accounts of abortion trail activism

Many Irish women are forced to come to Britain to obtain an abortion, as it's almost impossible to obtain one in Ireland, north or south. Large numbers come to Liverpool – it's nearest and has a [British Pregnancy Advisory Service] nursing home. They are faced with a long boat journey and the costs, not only of the abortion (over £100 now) but also for travel and accommodation for one night (another £50). Many women are young and travel alone on the board which has no medical facilities.

The boat arrives at approximately 6.30am and the women have to wait until the clinic opens at 10.00am. After they've met the counsellor, had an examination and spoken to the doctors, if an abortion is agreed to on both sides, the woman is given an appointment at the [British Pregnancy Advisory Service] nursing home in Parkfield Road for the night. They spend the next day and night in the nursing home, and are discharged at 8am the following morning; the boat leaves at 9 pm that evening.

Liverpool Abortion Support Service founding document,
Liverpool Central Archives

La primera red que se crea es la red de socorristas en red que abortamos. Que fue en el 2012 y que básicamente son compañeras que acompañaban de manera sorora aquellas mujeres y otras personas con capacidad de gestar que quisieran abortar consiguiéndoles misoprostol.

The first network created was the network of the Socorristas En Red Que Abortamos. That was in 2012 and they basically are compañera

who accompany in a <<sorora>> way those women and other pregnant people who wanted to abort using misoprostol.

Interviewee B202, Argentinian activist [author translation]

we were like 'oh my God, we can't believe that women die and there's the pill that does something'. We were shocked that, you wondered if the doctors know this, why don't they tell any . . . like, like this knowledge is available, the pills, because we started all to do like our own guerrilla warfare of going to clinic after clinic and asking and trying to buy the pills ourselves. [. . .] We found that a lot of pharmacists carried these pills, we, like it really shocked us that in our lifetime no-one had ever said this, like how is this a well-kept secret in this way? So, we immediately thought every woman should know this; how do we get out there and tell them? So, we started in our own small ways where plans could allow to go outside of Nairobi into rural areas and conducting this exact same training [. . .] We did not even make materials for this; we just took the training document from [organisation] we were trained with and just like repeated at that training over and over. Of course, there are challenges of how far you can go with that kind of strategy, but I would say we kept on say doing our best, and sort of using the 'train the trainers' model, and sort of trying to build like a whisper network.

Interviewee E109, sexual and reproductive health/self-managed abortion activist, Africa

Because, people who don't know their rights, they just assume, ok then, I have to pay. And if someone at reception, someone calls reception and says hey, this is my situation, and they tell them, ok that is 650 euros. They just hang up and they have a baby. This is something that we found out by a lot of research, speaking Dutch of course, which is also a big privilege of course, knowing the law, being able to read the law, knowing where to get it and so on and so forth. And most of the people that would want to get a free abortion in the Netherlands and are entitled to it, they will just simply not get to [have one] [if] they call a clinic that tells them they are not liable for a free abortion. And it took us maybe a year to realise that this is the law, after we started the group because nobody talks about this.

Interviewee TN101, abortion activist, the Netherlands

Four excerpts, from different contexts, located in different histories and parts of the world, with different strategies. The first, an excerpt from the founding document of the small collective based in Liverpool – the Liverpool Abortion Support Service (LASS) – was established to support abortion travel across borders. They were working with a well-known and well-worn abortion trail. As an Irish abortion activist based in Northern Ireland commented in another interview, the phenomenon of 'taking the boat to Liverpool' was something she was aware of as a child. They were also working within a jurisdiction where abortion had been liberalized over a decade previously through the passage of the Abortion Act 1967.

LASS was established when the process of accessing abortion in Liverpool was predominantly a surgical experience. This was an effect of both regulation and the willingness of public health services in Liverpool to provide abortion care. The promise of liberalization had not extended to Liverpool as much as feminist activists such as the Merseyside Abortion Campaign wished – press reports from the same period described Liverpool as one of the hardest places to access abortion through the UK's public health system (the National Health Service) – even though the legal framework permitted abortion. There were private clinics, including the British Pregnancy Advisory Service (BPAS), more than willing to provide abortion. However, as an effect of section 1 of the Medicines Act 1968, the use of medicines like mifepristone (RU486) was primarily restricted to NHS hospitals and BPAS required patients to book the day before the procedure took place and attend post-abortion care the following day.

The political context of the 1980s in Ireland, including but not limited to the politics of abortion, and the infrastructures of travel between the island of Ireland and Liverpool are also relevant to understanding LASS. Ferries were the main form of travel as the number of flights between Ireland and Liverpool were limited (six per week from Dublin – none on Mondays or Fridays – and four from Belfast). While the Eighth Amendment, the constitutional provision which recognized the 'unborn' as a rights-bearing citizen and acted as a de facto abortion ban, was not introduced until 1983 (four years after LASS was established), speakers from the Association for a Women's Right to Choose who attended the 1981 All-Ireland Women's Conference claimed that there was no abortion provision in either Northern Ireland or the Republic of Ireland. Unplanned pregnancy and the exercise of reproductive autonomy were restricted through a combination of social stigma. A carceral network of Mother and Baby Homes and Magdalene Laundries actively policed reproductive decision-making (McGettrick et al., 2021). It was not unusual for women to hide a pregnancy (Conlon, 2006), 'keep it secret' (Murphy Tighe and Lalor, 2016; Fletcher, 1995) or to take an impromptu visit to see an aunt abroad (Earner-Byrne and Urquhart, 2019). Although the island of Ireland was part of a Common Travel Area with England and Northern Ireland was part of the UK, the heightened political conflict and paramilitary attacks in England by terrorist organizations in Northern Ireland had resulted in the border between the two countries becoming increasingly securitized from the mid-1960s onwards (Hillyard, 1992), a point raised by Rossiter in her accounts of how the London-based Irish Women's Abortion Support Group assisted Northern Irish women travelling for abortion in *Ireland's Hidden Diaspora* (2009).

Information about abortion was scarce (Barry, 1988), a situation worsened by anti-choice campaigning agencies like the Society for the Protection of the Unborn Child pursuing information providers through the courts (Smyth, 2017). The limited information available was largely produced by feminist activist groups like the Women's Information Network (WIN) and circulated through informal channels or networks (Connolly, 1995) operating at the peripheries of the lawful (Cloatre and Enright, 2017). Activists in Ireland – North and South – had collaborated to disseminate information about where and how to access services in cities like Liverpool. Organizations like Open Line Counselling and the Irish Family Planning Association and activist networks like the Women's Information Network and the Ulster Pregnancy Advisory Agency provided information on clinic names and non-directive counselling. However, throughout the 1980s information providers, particularly in the Republic of Ireland, became subject to increasing control and were the target of anti-choice interventions. These include successive High Court challenges against the provision of information by and the existence of Open Door/Line Counselling by the Society for the Protection of the Unborn Child (SPUC). Within this environment, the ability of individual abortion seekers to learn the specifics of abortion access abroad was heavily curtailed.

Cumulatively, these contextual factors orientated LASS towards practical support work such as transport, accompanying, and hosting. They provided emotional support and reassurance but were not counsellors and did not offer post-abortion care. They collected abortion travellers from Liverpool port and arranged transport between clinics. They sat in waiting rooms alongside abortion seekers and provided somewhere to stay, a meal, and privacy. They provided activists in Ireland with a contact phone number and the name of a LASS member. These details were published by groups such as the Dublin Abortion Information Campaign, the Cork Abortion Information Campaign and the Students' Unions. Their main objective, according to interview data with activists as well as archival documents from the time, was to ameliorate the emotional, logistical and financial burdens facing women travelling from Ireland as well as partially normalize or, at least, destranger abortion (Fletcher, 2016; Duffy, 2020). For the majority of volunteers for these organizations, this was as far as their contribution went. As a member of LASS described:

> the help that we gave was mainly being available to go and pick up the girl or the woman at the ferry port if that was needed, sometimes women made their own way and we would get a phone call [. . .] but it was mainly the ferry port. When we met up our piece was just to give them a bed for the night, a meal, and just to be a listening ear. [. . .] It was really the practical things we did, when you're on a limited budget, not having to spend money on a B&B or a hotel is really important. (LASS 14)

The second comment is from an interview with an Argentinian feminist activist who had been involved in the campaigns for liberalizing, and ultimately decriminalizing, abortion legislation since the early 2000s. In this interview, the respondent spoke about the emergence of the *Ni Una Menos* (not one more) campaign and the *Marea Verde* (Green Wave) that has traversed Latin America and the Caribbean over the last ten to fifteen years and led to the liberalization and decriminalization of abortion access in countries such as Argentina, Chile, Uruguay and Colombia (Palmeiro, 2018). In Argentina, the *Socorristas en Red (Feministas que Abortamos)* are the best known feminist collective to self-identify themselves as supporting abortion seekers (Burton, 2017). The *Socorristas* adopt a networked structure, with local collectives across Argentina adopting the same practices, strategies and imagery.

As Maffeo et al. (2015) indicate, from their inception, the Socorristas explicitly aligned themselves to specific strategies and principles of reproductive politics. As the interviewee explains, the Socorristas engage in two key practices. Feminist accompaniment – as *compañeras* or *acompañante* activists – and information provision in public spaces and, for those who decide to have an abortion, in supportive conversations where they clarified how to use misoprostol (Maffeo et al., 2015). However, these actions are underlined by a political ideology that sees the abortion process as something that needs to be returned to women in a way that it can be safely practised rather than made safer through ensuring women have abortions in clinical settings or under the directions of medics. The interviewee describes this ideology as '*un manera sorora*' – a term which does not readily translate to English – but Maffeo et al. (2015) discuss as rooted in the following logic:

> *Desde una ética feminista, pensamos la situación del aborto como un acontecimiento a nivel subjetivo y colectivo que habilita un movimiento de autorización. En este sentido, la decisión autónoma de abortar devuelve y/o reafirma la construcción de la propia autoridad interna (Lagarde, 2001a), en oposición a las pretensiones patriarcales que históricamente han querido monopolizar la autoridad sobre las mujeres como grupo humano y depositar las autorizaciones en otros externos – instituciones o figuras– que se presentan con mayor supremacía.*

> From a feminist ethic, we think of the situation of abortion as an event at a subjective and collective level that enables an authorization movement. In this sense, the autonomous decision to abort returns and/or reaffirms the construction of one's internal authority in opposition to the patriarchal claims which historically have wanted to monopolize authority over women as a group and deposit authorizations in other external institutions or figures that are presented with greater supremacy. (Maffeo et al., 2015: 223; author's translation)

Vacarezza and Burton (2023), alongside numerous commentators writing from Latin America and the Caribbean and outside, have detailed how the Argentinian *Socorristas en Red*, and similar mobilizations such as *Las Parceras* (Colombia) and *Con las Amigas y En La Casas* (Chile), have worked to establish information hotlines and a model of care (feminist accompaniment) to support women to use misoprostol safely. These groups, many of which have mobilized under the transcontinental banner of *Red Compañera* since 2018, offer support through a combination of pedagogy and communication. They did not need to generate abortion trails – access routes to *pastillas* (abortion pills) as well as *yerberas* (herbal medicines) were well established before the *Socorristas en Red* self-identified as feminists who abort. The *Socorristas* emphasized this point in their organizing principle – '*las mujeres abortamos, las socorristas acompañamos* (women abort, socorristas accompany). However, these trails, in Argentina before the legalization of abortion in 2020 and in countries such as Peru, Paraguay, Honduras and parts of Mexico, have frequently operated clandestinely (Duffy, Freeman and Rodríguez, 2023). Women who have used them have faced harsh repercussions from state agencies. These risks, as Erdman, Jelinska and Yannow (2018) note, result in an environment where the experience of abortion is frequently unsafe, taking place in secrecy and under potentially harmful and risky conditions. Abortion trails' secrecy and clandestine nature have also reinforced abortion stigma and the marginalization of abortion from the public eye. Vacarezza and Burton (2023) argue that the result is an affective experience which lacks dignity.

Understanding the *Socorristas* requires contextualization within the broader gendered and reproductive politics in Argentina and Latin America and the Caribbean. Argentina, like other Latin American countries, has well-documented histories of gender-based violence (de Sousa and Rodrigues Selis, 2022), including reproductive harms, committed by State institutions and medical professionals, despite these institutions' claims, articulated through constitutional prohibitions on obstetric violence for example, to protect reproductive rights (Morgan and Roberts, 2012; O'Brien and Rich, 2022). Indeed, addressing the multiple forms of gender-based violence present in Argentina, including unsafe abortion, sexual violence, domestic violence and abuse and feminicide, was a core objective of the *Ni Una Menos* movement – which the *Socorristas* were part of (Daby and Moseley, 2022).

In terms of reproductive politics, the *Socorristas*, and Latin American abortion trail activism more generally, operate against a backdrop of uneven political economies of health and a promotion of contraception and improving birth outcomes or reducing maternal mortality rates above other forms of reproductive health care. Health policy research has highlighted the increased emphasis on establishing neoliberal, privatized and insurance-based health infrastructures in countries like Argentina over the course of the twentieth century (Segura-Ubiergo, 2007). For those reliant on public health systems, access was limited to centres which may or may not provide abortion. In the same period, progressive reproductive health policy in Latin America was conflated with expansive contraceptive access and addressing maternal mortality through improving care for mothers (Morgan, 2017).

Within this policy discourse, anti-abortion and restrictive reproductive policy gained further traction as a resolution to a gendered public health crisis, justifying at best policy apathy and at worst draconian legislation to prevent abortion. Morgan (2017) outlines how anti-abortion actors mobilized within the gendered health care and health policy space to reinforce the real problem as a lack of consideration for (potential) mothers, undermining any movement or even acceptance that abortion should be supported as a key form of reproductive health. The upshot in real terms was high rates of unsafe abortion and uneven access depending on class and income. Moreover, abortion seekers were cast as having failed to act as responsible reproductive citizens for not using contraception (De Zordo, 2016). Feminist activists combatted these problems through exploring safe, low-cost abortion methods which could exist outside the purview of the State. The most notable of these was the repurposing of misoprostol, originally licensed to treat stomach ulcers, as an abortifacient by Brazilian activists in the late 1990s. As it was already on the market, misoprostol was a low-cost, but ultimately, safe method. Although access to health care facilities was desirable, it was not essential, and abortion seekers could self-manage their health care outside clinical settings which were subject to state surveillance. Importantly, because they could avoid encounters with state institutions and could abort in privacy, the need to explain their decision-making or beg forgiveness for failing to manage their reproductive health responsibly was removed. That said, the growth of self-management expanded the regulatory terrain beyond prohibiting abortion access towards punishing those who presented with real or suspected post-abortion complications (De Zordo, 2016; Duffy, Freeman and Rodríguez, 2023).

This reality has influenced the work of *socorrisma* which aims not just to reduce the potential of harmful encounters through practical tactics – 'hot maps' of pharmacies and conscientious providers, information hotlines for pre- and post-abortion care, disseminating infographics on how to take misoprostol through social media – but to improve the experience of abortion. Part of the *Socorristas'* work involves moving abortion from the margins of reproductive health and creating an infrastructure of care where abortion seekers' experience is not determined by their economic status, where they do not have to ask permission or request care within a clinical setting, and where their right to privacy and autonomy will be respected. Moreover, *Socorristas* underlined the necessity for an infrastructure which actively respected abortion, as opposed to treating abortion as a failure to implement or comply with contraceptive policy successfully. While abortion should not happen clandestinely or treated as something that needs to be kept secret, individual privacy, dignity and autonomy should be respected. Abortion seekers should not rely on the state to condone or justify their actions.

The third comment at the beginning of this chapter is from an activist in Africa, working with an organization in 2003. In their interview, this activist relayed their experience establishing an infrastructure which could support access to safe, self-managed abortion using abortion pills. Initially working at a national level, with a focus on expanding knowledge and access to rural communities outside the major urban centres, the interviewee outlined how their organization had subsequently become part of a transnational network – the MAMA network. MAMA connects feminist collectives across Africa. Founded in 2016 it first had thirty member groups, predominantly in sub-Saharan Africa. This has since expanded and now includes members across the continent. The primary work of the interviewee's national feminist collective and the MAMA network focuses on providing information about abortion and sexual and reproductive health care through a helpline and online webchat facility, providing information about using abortion pills through sharing infographics on social media (specifically Twitter/X), and outreach work with rural communities to develop networks of community health leaders able to support the use of abortion pills and normalize abortion care.

What is interesting about the comments from this interviewee is that, even though she spoke of how she first learned about self-managed abortion using abortion pills and framed the work of her organization as innovative, she also noted that when they began to speak with communities they realized that local-level abortion trails already existed. Despite, from their perspective, the reticence of feminist movements in Africa to discuss abortion openly and a significant degree of abortion stigma and silencing, during discussions with community leaders and local women they heard numerous stories of abortion and local abortion care providers. As the interviewee commented:

> Because what we realised is that even when we are afraid of talking about abortion, almost in all communities if you spoke about it somebody knew someone [. . .] most likely an unsafe service. Like most likely it was a quack doctor. (E109, abortion activist, Africa)

As another activist within the broader network explained:

> but of course there are means that have always been done traditionally, you've go to these women, they give you these concoctions and then you swallow what they give you. The pregnancy is induced but not entirely, you know. There's a lot of complications and there are so many young women that are dying from it. (E202, abortion activist)

A priority of this network became communicating information publicly which could stabilize abortion trails, reduce the risk of encountering a 'quack doctor' and improve awareness of safe abortion methods. The interviewee detailed how their organization took a conscientious decision to develop a social media profile and set up a publicly advertised information phonelines in 2012. At the same time, they worked closely with communities, community leaders and grassroots networks to broaden awareness of safe abortion methods. They also undertook what the interviewee described as a 'guerrilla campaign', where they contacted pharmacists and health providers to try to access abortion pills themselves. This form of 'secret shopper' activity enabled them to locate access points for abortion pills as well as establish issues of cost and provider willingness to sell pills knowing that they would be put to this purpose.

Within communities, these activists engage in work that was more intimate and involved collective conversations, first about sexual and reproductive health and the rights of women and girls, before introducing unsafe abortion and abortion experiences to the conversation. The objective here was to, in the interviewee's words, 'change the narrative' around abortion as 'most of what we had in terms of people's experiences of abortion were harmful, self-harm sometimes, and unsafe'.

Through small-group conversations with women in communities, the interviewee's organization tried to draw attention to how common unsafe abortion experiences were, highlighting the need to openly discuss abortion, and then progressing the conversation to the ways that abortion safety could be improved – specifically through the use of abortion pills and supported self-management. This interviewee's group, and comparable national-level organizations across Africa, also worked with health providers, including community health workers and pharmacists. They began to hold sessions to clarify what the legal framework on abortion permitted, what safe abortion involved and how clinicians could address abortion stigma.

Again, the emphasis of this organization's work needs to be contextualized. They work within a regional context where liberalization of abortion access is ongoing, with many countries still operating under or tackling the legacies of restrictive legislation. For example, abortion was only affirmed as a human right under the Kenyan constitution in 2010. Historically, abortion has been criminalized except in emergency circumstances, where doctors feel continued pregnancy presents a risk to health or life of the mother. This historic criminalization has impacted the lived interpretation of abortion law by state officials, a dissonance between legal rights what Elwick describes as legal consciousness or perceptions about what the law says. Despite the Kenyan High Court's 2010 affirmation of abortion as a constitutional right and subsequent directive that parliament needed to enact reforms, as the Center for Reproductive Rights noted in 2022, 'women, girls and health care providers face harassment and intimidation'. The 2010 constitutional affirmation has been misinterpreted at a regional level with providers and abortion seekers targeted by police, a situation which led to the imprisonment of a minor and a clinician in 2020 in the town of Malindi, in the county of Kilifi, a county over 500 kilometres east of Nairobi and 80 kilometres north of Mombasa. The Center for Reproductive Rights and Reproductive Health Network Kenya (RHNK) submitted a complaint against officials in Malindi and Kilifi on behalf of the minor and clinicians to the Kenyan High Court. In the judgement – *PAK and*

Salim Mohammed v. Attorney General et al – the High Court reaffirmed their 2010 position on the fact that abortion was a human right and criminalization was an impairment of constitutional rights.

Organizations in the African space, such as the interviewee's, are also often established within the context of gross health inequities, with poorer and rural communities systemically disadvantaged in terms of both the availability of facilities and the cost of health care. As Chuma and Okungu (2011) outline in the Kenyan context, many African nations have regressive health financing systems due to a reliance on individual or out-of-pocket payments for health care to subsidize an under-funded public health system and an expanding, high-cost private health system. One off treatments in public health settings require individual additional payments, meaning those who require regular care but do not have private health cover (i.e. poorer communities) end up paying more for their health care than their wealthier peers. The health service network itself is also fragmented, with public care facilities offering a reduced range of services than private care centres.

For those in rural and isolated areas, these sorts of inequitable health systems create additional cost burdens related to travel. The interviewee recounted the problematic, and inequitable, economies of health based on conversations with rural communities in their country:

> Because even when we tried to share 'oh but there must be a place where there's services' and everyone was like 'yes, but it's 10,000/-', like 10,000/- to go and access that service. (E109, abortion activist Africa)

The interviewee's organization also needs to be discussed within the context of feminist activism in Africa at the present moment. The use of organizational information hotlines and social media is particularly pertinent here. As Nyabola (2018) writes, 'being feminist in Kenya can be dangerous' (p261). Individuals who make themselves visible as feminist activists are 'routinely ridiculed by both women and men' (Nyabola, 2018). Yet, despite the tendency of political analysts in Kenya and globally to label online feminist mobilizations as 'slacktivism' or ineffective, new media has given new voice to feminist concerns and allowed new, issue-based networks to coalesce, giving young radical feminists in particular a platform to push dialogue forward. (Nyabola, 2018: 262)

Within an environment where feminists, particular those involved in pro-abortion organizing, may face public shaming (as feminists) and institutional targeting by police services (as abortion advocates) and where online media has become an increasingly important space for reinforcing issue-based networks, establishing an information hotline and social media communication strategy is a logical strategic step.

The fourth and final comment is from an activist based in the Netherlands. Their organization, initially established to provide information and logistical support to those who had travelled to the Netherlands to access abortion services, had increasingly become involved in escorting abortion seekers to ensure their legal rights were respected and providing financial support to fully or partially cover abortion costs. The organization was principally based in Amsterdam but they actively collaborate with similar networks across Europe. They maintained an online presence, promoting their contact details through social media and providing an information helpline supported by volunteers who spoke English, Dutch and Polish. The context of abortion politics in Europe also orientated the actions of this interviewees group. The decision to look for volunteers for information helplines fluent in Polish and to share their contact details with Polish feminist networks was based on the increasingly restrictive legislative environment in Poland with regard to abortion access. This also influenced their movement towards acting as an abortion fund, as the interviewee recounted:

> We started off as just like a network that would basically erm help arrange procedures at the clinic, maybe translation and also arrange, erm, housing if needed for the time of the procedure here, but very quickly we realised people travelling from Poland cannot afford an abortion here because abortion in the Netherlands is interesting. It has basically one of the highest, legal limits to having an abortion

in the Netherlands is higher than all other European countries. Since UK is going to step out of EU. Erm, so it is 22 weeks and that means that a lot of people anyway, people from different countries travel to the Netherlands if pregnancy is above 12 or 16 weeks which is most countries in Europe. So getting a second trimester abortion which is anything between 18-22 weeks costs around 900 euros in the Netherlands and you can imagine erm yeah in Poland that can be to some people 2 monthly salaries. So yeah, very quickly we kind of realised, yeah, like erm a bottleneck. For a lot of people to get an abortion is to be able to afford it in the Netherlands so we started organising around gathering money basically to pay for at least a part of the procedure or the whole procedure. So now we are also a fund.

TN101 abortion activist, the Netherlands

The interview was conducted in June 2020, in the midst of the Covid-19 lockdowns, and so the interviewee said they were not currently offering hosting arrangements or transport to clinics but they had done so in the past.

The interviewee's comments are interesting and reflective of the legal and political context within which the organization emerged. The Netherlands has some of the most liberal abortion laws globally. In Europe it is a key destination for abortion travel from liberal and restrictive regimes due to the availability of later-gestation abortion care. The two largest transnational distribution networks for abortion pills – Women on Web and Women Help Women – were also founded in and continue to operate from the Netherlands. The interviewee's organization was therefore established in a country which has an established profile as a destination point and starting point for well-developed abortion trails involving abortion travel (to the Netherlands from liberal and illiberal abortion regimes) and distribution of abortion pills. However, while the legal permissibility of abortion in the Netherlands is regularly communicated, from the perspective of the interviewee, the sharing of information on health access policies, particularly relating to payment requirements, has not been discussed as openly with either abortion seekers or health care administrators. Research on migrant health in the Netherlands further notes that Dutch-language proficiency and knowledge of the Dutch health system may be significant barriers to accessing health care (Boateng et al., 2012). As the interviewee notes, poor understanding of health entitlements and the cost of care creates a substantial problem for migrant abortion seekers who are resident in the Netherlands. For this reason, their organization has increased escorting or accompanying actions and liaising with clinics on behalf of abortion seekers. This adds a further layer to their work.

Abortion trail activism

Even in contexts where abortion has been the target of sustained legal and political challenges, as well as intense social stigmatization and discrimination by health professionals, women have continued to access abortion services. There are numerous personalized accounts (Delay and Sundstrom, 2022; Darcy, 2020), theatrical representations (O'Connor, 2015), films (Eliza Hittman's 2020 *Never Rarely Sometimes Always*), fictionalized accounts (e.g., Jenni Hendricks and Ted Kaplan's 2019 Young Adult novel *Unpregnant*) and media articles about historic and contemporary abortion access outside formal architectures of health care access. As the four opening accounts illustrate, for many, abortion access is facilitated by networks of activists operating around, or in direct contravention to, restrictions. These include anti-abortion regulations, structural inequalities in the availability of abortion services or the absence of access points for abortion.

As well as the cultural representations, there are now important scholarly interventions exploring the dynamics and lived realities of the collectives and networks facilitating abortion access, outside or in spite of prohibitions, from the perspective of activists (Rossiter, 2009), abortion seekers (Cohen and Joffe, 2020) and academics (Sethna and Davis, 2019; Calkin and Freeman, 2019; Coast et al., 2018). These pathways to abortion are frequently clandestine (Duffy, Freeman and

Rodríguez, 2023), complex and financially burdensome (Kimport, 2022; Coast et al., 2021) as well as personally isolating. Some scholars represent these infrastructures as State-sanctioned banishment (Erdman, 2016), that they are produced by fundamentally disciplinary reproductive frameworks and should thus be interpreted as 'medical tourism' by coercion rather than choice (Bloomer and O'Dowd, 2014; Sethna and Doull, 2012).

The field of reproductive justice and abortion scholarship is witnessing a burgeoning body of research and writing on the actors, and practices of these actors, that support and shape the experience of accessing abortion outside the State. This includes analysis of historic and contemporary movements assisting travel across and within countries (Sethna and Davis, 2019; Sethna and Doull, 2012), networks which distribute abortion pills and construct maps of points of access (Calkin and Freeman, 2019; Veldhuis, Sánchez-Ramírez and Darney, 2022a), organizations providing financial support such as the US National Network of Abortion Funds and UK Abortion Support Network (Fried, 2013; Bloomer, Pierson and Estrada, 2018), and lay 'abortion doulas' offering pre- and post-abortion care (Campbell et al., 2021).

Collectively, this literature challenges certain media representations of the networks of actors that facilitate abortion access within restrictive legal regimes or where a combination of social stigma, concerns of encountering judgemental health professional attitudes, provider reluctance or objection to engaging in abortion care, or inadequate financing result in abortion-seeking outside the State. Rather than replicating depictions of these abortion pathways as inherently risky, backstreet or only utilized out of desperation (Assis and Erdman, 2022), academics and members of organizations themselves highlight the coherence and sophistication of the 'constellation of actors' (Berro Pizzarossa and Nandagiri, 2021). Furthermore, this body of writing highlights the role of these actors in transforming the affective experience of abortion (Vacarezza and Burton, 2023), addressing abortion stigma (Drovetta, 2020) and advancing health technologies, specifically telehealth and telemedicine. Connectedly, there is an emerging discussion of the contribution of these networks to improving abortion care or how their practices can be mirrored by new formal or State-sanctioned abortion care infrastructures (McReynolds-Pérez et al., 2023).

At the same time, the global conversation about the historic and contemporary infrastructures of abortion access – a theoretical frame that refers to the diverse practices, objects, actors and things that enable people to meet their daily needs (Alam and Houston, 2020; Furlong, 2011) – draws attention to its undeniable diversity. Simply put, there is no one type, and certainly no single transferrable type, of network supporting abortion access outside the State, in restrictive or fragmented abortion care regimes. Entering this terrain, one could easily get quickly bogged down in describing the differences between movements. Such descriptive labour also presents potential risks, not least the risk of overlooking the increasingly recognized similarities between movements in very different spaces and places (Braine and Velarde, 2022). Furthermore, as writing on social movement studies more broadly indicates, description can result in the application of broad distinctions between what counts as 'true' activism (Bobel, 2007), which exclude the contributions directed at quotidian, lived experiences of reproductive injustice that form the core intervention of key abortion activists and mobilizations (Duffy, 2020; Ruibal and Fernadez Anderson, 2020).

To avoid such pitfalls, this volume begins by accepting the nebulousness of the shape, structure, size and activities that form the basis of the networks supporting abortion access outside of a 'formal' architecture of abortion care provision. To emphasize this point, I discuss them under the heading of abortion trail activism. The term trail held a particular attraction as it partly defies a specific interpretation. In his 2016 part-autobiographical, part-analytical work *On Trails*, the travel writer Robert Moor explores both the 'soul' and realities of trails. Moor's reflections are based on his experience of first walking and then working on the Appalachian Trail. In his far-reaching discussion, Moor argues that while there are very physical and visible characteristics of the Appalachian Trail, it is much more than a connection of material objects writing that

> [T]he soul of a trail – its *trail-ness* – is not bound up in dirt and rocks; it is immaterial, evanescent, as fluid as air. (Moor, 2016: 2)

What is significant about Moor's analysis is not just its aspiration to move trails from the 'periphery of our gaze' (Moor, 2016) to the centre of a sustained discussion but the fact that it does not offer a straightforward understanding of what a trail is. *On Trails* does not explain what trails are. Where explanations are presented, they are contradictory. For example, while Moor's text defines by functionality, stating that trails 'persist because they connect one node of desire to another' and disappear 'once the desire fades' (p3), this statement does not accurately reflect *On Trails*' contentions about the realities of trails. There is no *need* for the Appalachian Trail from a purely functional perspective. If trails naturalistically fade as the need for them is removed, then why are there organizations – which Moor himself has collaborated with – actively working to conserve trails which arguably are no longer necessary?

One reason for the persistence of trails after they are necessary is offered by analyses of urban ecologies and mobilities – from architecture, urban planning, transport, anthropology and geography. An established trope within writing in relation to urban space (physical and social) is an appropriation of what Bachelard labelled *les chemins du désir* or desire lines (Bachelard, 2014 [1957]; see: Furman, 2012). The brief definition is that desire lines or desire paths are the visible trails, tracks and cut-throughs that occur as the *users* of urban spaces *move within* urban spaces. As Luckert (2012) writes in her cartographical analysis of desire lines in Edmonton (Canada), 'desire lines are unsanctioned paths worn only by frequent footsteps' (p. 318).

However, successive analyses of desire lines do not reinforce such a succinct definition. Like trails, a purely functional reading of desire lines does not offer a comprehensive insight into their essence. As Luckert alludes, desire lines are also historical records and exist in memory as much as in lived urban cartographies. Focusing on Cape Town, Murray et al. offer a more expansive reading of desire lines arguing that these paths

> indicate the space between the planned and the providential, the engineered and the 'lived', and between the official projects of capture and containment and the popular energies which subvert, bypass, supersede and evade them. (Murray, Shepherd and Hall, 2007: 1)

This interpretation of desire lines suggests that they are not just dynamic in the sense that they emerge continuously due to movement, but also in the sense that they reflect the relationship between 'officialdom' and the public. A similar vision of desire lines is presented by Luckart's colleague Perkins (Luckert, 2012) who conceptualizes these urban trails as collective communication – the mechanism through which the public provide feedback to urban planners and officials. Importantly, this feedback is not just about what the public want or need in terms of the movement through urban space; desire lines have also been presented as spatial articulations of resistance and reclamations of space by the public. Indeed there is writing in political geography positioning desire lines as a manifestation of collective socio-spatial dissent to restrictive and defensive architectures within urban spaces used by the State to regulate how and under what conditions public space can be used (Smith and Walters, 2018).

Moor's trail imagining and desire lines share a number of characteristics. Both emphasize collective engagement and the fact that trails and desire lines are dynamic. The outsideness – physical and metaphorical – of both trails and desire lines are underlined in literature. Even in literature focused on desire lines *within* urban spaces, such as shopping malls and urban filaments between and within buildings (Furman, 2012), these lines are conceptualized as exterior, albeit in this case exterior to the intentions of city planners. Furman's intervention is noteworthy as it distinguishes between desire lines and *sight lines*, reminding us again that visibility and seeing is not always a prerequisite of a desire line. As in the broader readings of Perkins and others on desire lines and the arguments of trail conservationists and users of the Appalachian Trail, while the *functional* need for these pathways may fade, their role as spatialized historical records and cultural artefacts may persist.

Interestingly, both trails and desire lines partially disrupt hierarchical interpretations of collective dissent, although admittedly desire lines more explicitly. Trails and desire lines become distinguishable because of collective rather than individual action. As Moor contends, while the trope of individual 'trailmakers' certainly exists in public consciousness, 'trail followers' are equally important to the operations and essence of trails. It is through the actions and participation of 'trail followers' that trails become more sophisticated, more expansive and more advanced. Similarly, while Bachelard first proposed desire lines as the result of individual yearning to move in a certain way in a cityscape, there is widespread recognition that there is no linear history of a desire line and their existence cannot be attributed to an individual.

Beyond desire lines, a further interpretation of trails is offered in discussions of border mobilities and security in East Africa through the figure of *panya* routes. *Panya* routes or 'rat' routes in Swahili are informal pathways used daily by those crossing borders within and between East African countries. *Panya* routes are particularly common along the largely porous Ugandan-Kenyan borders. Unlike desire lines, *panya* routes are not discussed in literature on trails or collective mobilities within lived spaces. For the most part *panya* routes are considered in writing on border securities and regulation. They are associated with a very different purpose than urban desire lines or hiking trails; *panya* routes are linked to illicit trading of arms and narcotics, human trafficking and guerrilla incursions. This link is not unwarranted – there are numerous accounts of criminal and violent experiences, including gender-based violence, along *panya* routes. Personal experiences of violence and *panya* travel are well documented in public hearings of the Truth, Reconciliation and Justice Commission of Kenya (TJRC, 2011). Jacques Pauw's 2012 work *Rat Roads* offers a vivid account of Kennedy

Gihana's use of *panya* routes to travel from Rwanda to South Africa in the aftermath of the 1994 Rwandan conflict. The criminal character of *panya* routes is further reinforced by the adoption of the name Panya Road by violent gangs in Dar es Salaam and Zanzibar (Mohamed and Mussa, 2019).

That said, *panya* routes are not purely criminal or violent pathways. There is substantial literature on the everyday use of *panya* roads by small traders on the Kenyan-Ugandan and Kenyan-Tanzanian borders. Indeed, in their analysis of border regulation and securitization at the Isebania border between Kenya and Tanzania, Maroa (2013) addresses *panya* routes in much more expansive terms. Maroa's description of *panya* routes (included below) is worth exploring in depth as it illustrates both the complexities of these trails and the resonances of the *panya* roads and less security-focused conceptualizations of desire lines and trails. As Maroa writes:

> Cross border women traders at the Isebania border of Kenya and Tanzania use the unofficial entry point commonly known as 'panya' routes which loosely translated into Kswahili means, 'rat route'. The panya route comprises a short-cut, usually a small path, commonly used by ordinary civilians living in an area to cross into either side of the two countries in the course of their daily business. In most instances Panya routes are of no concern to the border security officials and hence remain un-manned. They exist with tacit official approval, to facilitate the movement of ordinary permanent inhabitants of the border post area, who in most cases also have cross-border linkages when crossing the border, inhabitants of border posts exploit the 'freedom' that goes with panya routes, which constitute major conduit points for illicit trade not only in arms but also in Drugs, Foodstuffs, Human trafficking, Vehicle theft, Minerals and precious stones, Game trafficking and Money laundering. (Maroa, 2013: 41; capitalization in original)

Maroa's depiction of *panya* routes is significant for a number of reasons. First, while there is a clear statement that these routes are used for illicit activity and serious crime, the use of *panya* for 'ordinary' trading purposes by residents is given equal recognition. Second, Maroa presents *panya* routes and the use of these routes as outside officialdom but not invisible to officialdom. *Panya* routes may be unmanned but that does not necessarily mean they are hidden. Third, the description of *panya* roads suggests that, like Perkins' description of 'desire lines', these routes are intertwined with socio-spatial realities and historic experiences. Residents live across and along *panya* routes and have done so for some time. Fourth, Maroa openly associates *panya* route-usage with *women*.

What emerges from this reading of *panya* route travel is a much more complex imagining than a straightforward association of these roads with crime and violence. As well as being insecure, these paths are commercial and well trodden. They are also gendered and indicative of a transnational 'living' history of how informal trails persist to address material inequalities experienced by the most disadvantaged (Nakanjako, Onyango and Kabumbuli, 2021). Interestingly, while sexual violence along *panya* routes is well documented (Ashe and Ojong, 2022), there is also evidence indicating that women small traders use *panya* routes to avoid sexual harassment from border security (Ruiter, Hadley and Li, 2017). It is also worth noting that many known *panya* routes traverse borders which were imposed upon East Africa by Western colonialists. As Maroa notes, the communities regularly using *panya* roads are part of cross-border communities. This point is not unimportant as it raises the question of what is 'outside' – the *panya* route or the 'legal' border.

Maroa is not alone in raising the complex, historically entrenched, and gendered nature of *panya* routes and route-usage. Tamale (2020), for example, proposes that *panya* travel arguably reflects the fact that "African *wananchi*[1], in their day-to-day existence, hardly respect the made-in-Berlin borders" (Tamale, 2020: 368). She notes that the celebrated Pan-Africanist advocate Tajudeen Abdul-Raheem provokes

---

[1] Hswahili for the ordinary people; the public – refers to East African communities.

a similar reading of *panya* routes, suggesting that those who use *panya* roads are simply acting as 'good Pan-Africanists'. Moreover, as in Maroa's reflection of *panya* route-usage and commerce, the fact that these roads are predominantly used by women small traders is emphasized in studies of East and sub-Saharan African economies (Tamale, 2020; Tsikata, 2009; Darkwah, 2007). The gendered use of *panya* routes is explored by academic research on the informal economy and the effect of the regulation of commodities trade as part of the reinforcement of the historically porous Kenyan-Ugandan, as well as the regulation and imposition of trade borders more generally, by political elites (national and international). While the dangers of *panya* trails is made explicit, so too are the vested interests behind the eradication of these trails by States seeking to reclaim the financial benefits of micro- and informal trade. The writing on *panya* also recognizes their generative potential for communities most subject to State discrimination, including migrants and women.

Read alongside each other, desire lines analyses, the Global North trail writing of Moor and *panya* road discussions appear to offer vastly different definitions of trails. At face value, desire lines/trails and *panya* routes are incomparable. Literature on desire lines and trails makes no reference to the use of these passageways as facilitating violent crime or the types of illicit activities framed as inherent components of *panya* roads. Even where desire lines are positioned as resistant or representations of political dissent, they are separated from more 'serious' crimes such as arms smuggling, the drugs trade or human trafficking. Where danger or threat is explored in literature on desire lines, the discussion focuses on the threat of repercussions from 'above' rather than threats within the paths themselves. Similarly, as Stanley (2020) notes in his analysis of hiking, trail usage is almost always associated with positive aspirations, a source of 'redemption, enjoyment, meaning, and challenge' (Stanley, 2020: 241). Despite the fact that both rural and urban trails in the Global North are used for the movement of narcotics, sexual exploitation and human trafficking (McLean, Robinson and Densley, 2019; Moyle, 2019), these features of trails receive little-to-no attention in Moor's trail writing or desire line conceptualizations influenced by Bachelard.

On the other hand, outside of work on the gendered usage of *panya* routes in the informal economy and Tamale's provocation as to whether these roads should be read as feminist, literature considering *panya* roads in the tones used in trail- and desire line-writing is almost non-existent. *Panya* road travel is always dangerous. As Ashe and Ojong's and Tsikata's work makes abundantly clear, the nuances of quotidian *panya* route-taking, the histories of *panya* routes and their contribution to individual and collective economic well-being are marginalized within conversations about political liberalization and contemporary African transnational policy. The fact that informal traders, who are predominantly women, opt to continue to use *panya* routes to avoid interactions with State infrastructures as the latter are not always harmless or benevolent actors, can be missed by a lumpen treatment of *panya* as dangerous.

My aim here is not to say that all trails are equal – there are differences between hiking trails, urban cut-throughs and cross-border routeways that are regularly used for arms and narcotics trafficking. What I want to draw attention to is the *tonal* difference in how we speak, write and think about the routeways that fall under the broad umbrella of trail. I want to provoke a more active reflection on the relatively liberal use of the word 'informal' in conversations about trails as well as what scrutiny of these trails can tell us about the problems of formal passageways. I aim to draw attention to how significant the geographic location of both the trails and those theorizing trails is to our understanding of trails. As Luckert, Murray and others suggest, desire lines are a mix of spatiality, emotion and temporality. As such, the *where* of trails and the history of those places is significant. The tone with which trails are discussed depend on the place-history and place-memory.

It is important not to approach the politics of trails as a binary politics – either as dissent or functionalism – but as a form of politics which defies a static, fixed interpretation. As even a cursory comparison between different 'types' of trail illustrates, any one answer to the question 'what is a trail?' is going to be inevitably reductive and obscure critical important parts of the discussion. We are, arguably, never going to establish a single, satisfactory definition of 'a trail'. At this juncture, it also is worth noting that thus far I have focused on *physical* trails. In reality, these are just one 'type' of trail – information communication connections have also been addressed as trails or pathways for some time. Indeed, Claude Shannon (1993), one of the foremost innovators in cybernetics and information communication technologies, conceptualized his work as contributing to means for facilitating movement of data along channels.

Equally important is avoiding binary interpretations of trails as positive or negative. What the above section shows is that the affective experience of trails and the systems of power within them are inherently ambivalent. As writing on queerness and trails indicates, even the most official-looking 'safe' trail can be felt as exclusionary and disciplining. Social, cultural and embodied capital run through and shape the experience of trail-taking. The space is simply more accessible and welcoming to those who fall visibly into particular social and embodied categories. Furthermore, how trails are read – as safe, unsafe, acceptable or in need of eradication – is shaped by a combination of contextual factors (i.e. where they are and when they emerge) as well as their usage (including who uses them and for what purpose). The brief review above also shows the complex reasons why trails may be preserved, even when they present substantial dangers. This includes the potential for trail-takers to avoid the gaze of the State which, depending on their subjectivity and social position, is a persistently harmful actor.

As well as this, trail writing recognizes the differing roles of the actors connected to and within trails. Trail writing highlights that, regardless of the imagining in some bodies of literature of trail-taking as fundamentally an isolated experience (by trail blazers or people following lines of desire), actors linked to trails predominantly work collectively. The collective labour of trail workers includes repair and maintenance, as well as conservation and refinement. These labours are shaped by the orientation of trails towards utility as well as the understanding of trails as historical infrastructures and sites of collective memory. Significantly, the specific tasks that trail workers undertake to repair, maintain, conserve or refine trails are frequently small. If we imagine the everyday, small-scale work of clearing trails of debris or waste, these are undoubtedly minor actions when performed by individuals. However, as a collective enterprise they are essential to enabling the continued functioning of trails. It is also worth recognizing that trail workers may not always have shared goals or consistent ideas of what 'good' trail work should look like. Conservationists and those who work to maintain continuity of form or function may work at cross purposes by those who work to repair or update trails so they become more efficient and stable.

How trails are remembered, memorialized or retained is similarly complex. Trails sit within a colonialist legacy as well as a decolonial politics. Trails, including the Appalachian Trail that Moor waxes lyrical about, run alongside historical narratives of colonial violence. This includes sustained epistemic violence, where the sophistication and technologically advanced character of pre-colonial histories have been destroyed and erased (Vázquez, 2009) as part of colonial projects to present White European histories and knowledges as more progressive, refined and modern. It also involves the neocolonialist project of retaining control and supremacy over the Global South by the Global North through maintaining control over the means of production. Trail memorialization and retention is relevant to the neocolonialist project as one of the ways that the Global North prevents Global South countries from taking advantage of their natural resources or means of production comprehensively is through identifying spaces as sites of pilgrimage (Purnomo et al., 2022). The key issue here is what happens when trails are absorbed into formal national and transnational historiography and whether this enables additional technologies of control to circulate.

For me, trail is a useful way to emphasize the complexity of the networks of actors working on and supporting abortion access. The term accepts diversity of infrastructural form, organizational structure and types of work by those within these sites of activism. Equally, it offers a means of articulating these activisms in a way that appreciates their history and their status as a praxis engaged with a tangible object (a trail) that has been and continues to be collectively remade. Trails open discussions about narrative politics, foregrounding how presentation and framing of trails reflect preconceptions about the practices and qualities of health infrastructures outside a 'formal', officially sanctioned architecture that is subject to regulatory governance. The potential for trails to be treated in vastly different ways depending on who uses them, where and for what purposes is relevant to a conceptual discussion about the means of accessing abortion outside State- or medically sanctioned and managed routeways.

At the same time, trail analysis progresses from the expectation that there is, despite the differences between trails, broad similarities in their intent, role and position in comparison to formal infrastructures. Trails are intended to facilitate transport and movement. The label trail thus has analytic possibilities for querying the characteristics and benefits of 'formalized' abortion care. Under the parameters of trails, it is possible, and indeed desirable, to critically engage with what happens when abortion care and provision is absorbed by the State through liberalization or establishing sanctioned abortion trails. Trails can be useful to open space for articulating differing perspectives on what the orientation of the pro-choice abortion project is and reflecting on how narrative framings of 'unsanctioned' abortion access routes shape the pro-choice project towards potentially problematic goals.

The book proceeds from these considerations.

Structure of the book

The book is organized around two interventions, across five chapters, each of which contains a combination of primary data from activist organizations and references to sociological theory and existing literature on abortion activism, activist movements and abortion politics. The first intervention, which forms the first part of the book, aims to foreground abortion trail activism as a distinguishable political praxis. My objective here is to, on the one hand, identify the resonances across the various movements that I connect with in this form of activism globally and, on the other, provide a robust understanding of what characterizes this as a form of activism. The impetus for part one comes out of a recognition of the limited globally orientated writing attempting to connect movements in vastly different jurisdictions, but which are committed to similar aims, to a shared political ideology.

As already noted, there is a vibrant discussion within academic writing on abortion activism on practical support networks or abortion infrastructures outside the State as a feminist political force. This discussion has highlighted the role of these infrastructures in driving forwards progress on, for example, self-managed abortion and telemedicine. Since the early 2000s, there has been increasing attention paid to accompaniment abortion groups and networks – through *acompañante* movements – outside the State in the Latin American context as having distinguishable political commitments, commitments which are reflected in their core engagements. Prior to and alongside this scholarship, there is a substantial body of literature focused on abortion travel organizations and abortion funds, particularly in the Global North. This work has looked at, among other things, the role of activists in ameliorating the experiences of those living in restrictive legal environments forced to travel and the emotional support they offer to abortion seekers.

The problem, that this book aspires to provoke further consideration on, is whether this conversation can be expanded beyond regional parameters or clusters of organizing (i.e. *acompañante*, self-managed abortion activism, abortion funds, practical support for travel and so on). The first three chapters look at the shared commitments – manifesting in abortion trail activism – underpinning mobilizations of different size, in different jurisdictions, with varying localized concerns and contextual histories. Drawing on primary and archival research, these chapters present three characterizing features of abortion trail activism transnationally. These are concerns with accessibility (*Chapter 1*), to projecting a non-ontological reading of abortion according to feminist ethic of care principles (*Chapter 2*) and to pursuing a prefigurative politics which generates a transformative vision of what abortion care could look like in the present moment (*Chapter 3*). These chapters draw on a range of theoretical lenses related to care, access and prefiguration.

The book's second intervention, progressing through *Chapters 4 and 5*, is that looking directly at abortion trails is not just useful for showing the distinguishable political praxis that manifests in diverse ways, but also carries analytic benefits for scholarly conversations about the contradictions within pro-choice abortion politics. Here I want to focus on narrative politics and how the intent of the pro-choice project is shaped through framings of abortion trails. I am interested in how thinking critically on the varied ways abortion trails are framed, as is the case with the term trails, can make us more attentive to the contestations within narratives of pro-choice abortion politics' intent. Specifically, looking at the framing of abortion trails, we can see how the narrative of pro-choice abortion politics as involving a trend towards treating it through human rights' frameworks and promoting broader self-management and task sharing by non-clinically-trained health workers can be contested. In *Chapter 4* I present three distinguishable framings of abortion trails – as legally outside, as a lifeline and as a shadow infrastructure of abortion – which I then consider in *Chapter 5* as pointing to a persistent tension within the pro-choice abortion project between formalization of abortion access under a State-sanctioned governing architecture or preservation of abortion trails as non-normative, agile, and subject to ongoing remaking. Abortion trails are an apt mechanism for teasing out this tension. Like all trails, they continually bear witness to arguments regarding the need to maintain an unsanctioned, outside passageway, the benefits of making these passageways safer, and the risks of ceding or seeking control of trails by the State.

In Chapter 5 I discuss the problems that arise if the pursuit of pro-choice abortion politics is the formalization of abortion trails, using the examples of Ireland and Colombia, arguing that the formal abortion pathways constituted in these countries, designed to address the use of unsafe abortion trails outside the State, contain exclusions and lived barriers to abortion. Through this discussion, I note how the orientation towards formalization and State control has been legitimized through the narrative framings of abortion trails. This raises an important question regarding the contribution of abortion trails to the pro-choice abortion space and whether they prefigure alternatives to abortion care or legitimize the formation and imposition of a rigid, State and medical-institution-led framework of abortion care which is designed to address the 'negative' (i.e. dangerous) aspects of abortion trails.

The book's *Conclusion* restates the *Introduction*'s opening comments, which emerged from reflections on my own positionality and reproductive experiences as well as encounters with activist (Lord, 2013; Rosso, 2021), creative and scholarly (Jeppesen and Nazar, 2012) comments about the reality of getting an abortion and the importance of centring this experience in discussions on reproductive autonomy and choice. Drawing these reflections together with the theoretical frames applied in the book, the Conclusion argues that, despite the variations in specific movements, at different points in time, working in different jurisdictions, there are identifiable, shared commitments underpinning the organizations that support abortion trails. Moreover, it is clear from the comments of activists that they view their work as decidedly political, in a feminist and prefigurative sense. What we can draw from this is that abortion trail activism is not just a functional response but a specific, political interpretation of what abortion care should look like and what a feminist practice or infrastructure of abortion care should aim to do. Echoing its earlier arguments, the Conclusion underscores that centring abortion trails activism as political is also analytically important in terms of revealing the problematics within a pro-choice abortion project that pursues formalization of abortion care under the auspices of the State.

Methodology, positionality and language-use statement

This book is based on extensive primary research, in the form of over eighty semi-structured interviews (in-person, by telephone and by online video platform), desktop and archival research (in archives in Liverpool as well as activists' personal archives) over a seven-year period, beginning in 2016, as part of three interconnected but distinct research projects. The first of these – the *Liverpool Ireland Abortion Corridor: History, Activism and Health Care Practice* – was supported by Wellcome Trust Seed Grant in Humanities and Social Science and an interdisciplinary project involving researchers at Manchester Metropolitan University, University of Liverpool and Edge Hill University. The project focused specifically on the abortion trail between the island of Ireland and Liverpool, exploring the activist networks that supported abortion travellers to Liverpool as well as the effect on travel on health care giving and practice. The research was qualitative and archival, involving twenty-six semi-structured interviews with key informants in health care provision and abortion trail activism in the Republic of Ireland and Northern Ireland as well as archival research in Liverpool Central Library, Linen Hall Library Belfast, the Public Records Office of Northern Ireland and activists' personal archives. Interviews were conducted by phone or face to face by myself and the project research assistant (Dr Claire Pierson) working individually or together. The LIAC study resulted in one co-authored and one single-authored paper (Duffy et al., 2018; Duffy, 2020).

The second project – *Sexual and Reproductive Health and Rights in Colombia* – was a collaboration between two researchers in the UK (myself and Dr Megan Daigle) and an independent researcher who worked in Argentina and Colombia (Ms Diana López Castañeda). This project was supported by the two UK institutions (Manchester Metropolitan University and University of Birmingham) and involved thirty semi-structured interviews with activists, health policy makers, health care professionals and health service managers in Bogotá and

Cali. Interviews were all conducted in Spanish, with the researchers working in pairs. The project resulted in one co-authored journal article (Daigle, Duffy and Castañeda, 2022) and two amicus curiae briefs.

The third project – *Feminist Outlaws: Abortion Trail Activism and the Evolution of Pro-Choice Politics* – was a Fellowship project funded by the Leverhulme Trust. This project was originally designed to include substantial fieldwork in the United States, Ireland and Latin America. However, due to Covid-19 restrictions the project had to be adapted substantially. All semi-structured interviews (twenty-six in total) had to be conducted by online video platform or telephone. The location of interviewees also needed to shift due to the impact of different time zones. Following unsuccessful attempts to undertake interviews from the United Kingdom with participants based in Latin America and the United States, the research was redesigned to focus more actively on activists in Africa. This presented its own methodological challenges as abortion activists and feminist activists are at significant risk in this space, much more so than activists on the island of Ireland or the United States. To protect interviewees, the use of identifiers had to be kept to a minimum. The research was again collaborative – with one independent researcher and two other academics based, at time of research, in the United Kingdom and United States – with an understanding that parts of the dataset could be used in collaborators' own research. A co-authored article using data from activists in the African space is, at time of writing, under production.

The majority of interviews informing this monograph's analysis were conducted and transcribed, verbatim, in English. Those conducted in Spanish were transcribed in Spanish. Where interviews have been quoted in this book, the verbatim quote is presented in the original language with my own translation below. Where possible, quotes have been attributed to an organization or specific country. However, in some circumstances the attribution is more general to protect the participant.

Interview data analysis has been influenced by writing on thematic analysis, specifically reflexive thematic analysis (Braun and Clarke, 2019, 2021). Reflexive thematic analysis can arguably be read as a reinterpretation or less rigid articulation of thematic analysis as praxis rather than a fixed analytic framework. It emerged from critiques of thematic analysis, in the form outlined by Braun and Clarke (2006) as having "*codified* practice, prioritised procedure [. . .] and created rigid and concrete 'rules'" (Braun and Clarke, 2021: 329). Reflexive thematic analysis corrects the application of thematic analysis as a set of rules by presenting qualitative data analysis as a process of constructing arguments led by a combination of *inductive* reasoning grounded in data collected and *deductive* interpretation of data guided by other research and theories.

The reason I am identifying reflexive thematic analysis as important to this study at this point is to foreground that the readings presented in this volume are a product of my perspective (and therefore my positionality), the data I have gathered and the research and theoretical frames I have engaged with. Another researcher, not based in the Global North or sociology, who is not as connected personally to a country where abortion trail activism had featured so significantly in feminist history may have pursued or undertaken the same project in a very different way. There are conversations to be had about the potential divergences between the arguments I present here and those that a researcher based in the African, Latin American, North American, (mainland) European or South Asian space (for example) may have produced.

There are obvious limitations to this study, and important caveats. The data itself is limited and participants not evenly distributed. Recruitment was influenced by gatekeepers, existing networks and the effects of Covid-19 lockdowns on travel and face-to-face data collection. There are clearly numerous missing voices in this study and it would be incorrect to present it as the final word on abortion trail activism or even as comprehensively global in its representativeness or coverage. As a White, Global North academic in the Higher Education Institutions, there are limitations to my data collection capacities. I cannot speak for activists, as an activist, as a member of a Black Indigenous or People of Colour (BIPOC) community, as a member of the Latinx community or as someone with a physical impairment or learning disability. I cannot speak for a feminist living and working in a contested territory, in Latin America, Africa, North America, mainland Europe or Asia. I cannot speak as a health care provider.

As an additional point on language, in this volume, guided by the phrasing used by activists, I will use gendered terminology. I have tried to remain faithful to the terms interviewees' used as much as possible. That said, I do not use gendered terms ('women' 'girl') according to 'biological' interpretations of sex. The category 'women' in this work is inclusive and does not differentiate between trans* and non-binary communities. Similarly, at times I will use the short form names of countries. As such the terms 'Ireland' should be interpreted as the Republic of Ireland rather than the island of Ireland (which includes Northern Ireland) unless otherwise stated. Finally, I use the terms Global North and Global South. Global North is a political category, referring to the countries who have historically acted/continue to act as (neo)colonialist elites; Global South refers to countries historically and continually subject to exploitation by the Global North. Given that not all countries in the Global South geographically were or are colonial powers and communities within the Global North (such as indigenous and First Nations peoples) have extensive experiences of exploitation and colonial harms, these terms are potentially flawed categorizations. Alternative terms include minority (extractive, colonialist) and majority (exploited, colonized) worlds. I have opted not to use minority/majority for this volume – although I have used these terms elsewhere – as Global North/Global South is currently more recognizable within academic writing.

1

Access

Introduction

In this and the following chapter I want to outline an image of abortion trail activism as a manifestation of political praxis built around two main immediate concerns. By 'immediate' I mean the daily work that occupies activists within the abortion trail political space. These occupying concerns are what characterizes abortion trail activism. Here I address the first characteristic – addressing (in)accessibility. The chapter will adopt a health research lens and accessibility approach, considering access as 'the ability to derive benefits out of things' (Ribot and Peluso, 2003: 153). In doing so, I will propose the focal point of abortion trail activism – the problem it seeks to address – as the interface between the individual 'outside' the domain of health care and the 'point of entry' to getting care. The chapter will then illustrate how this orientation presents itself in the work of abortion trail activists by considering how they address three key barriers identified in writing on health accessibility – material, epistemic and cultural.

My observations in this and the following chapters are based on research on abortion trail activist movements, past and present, in a range of places globally. As a starting point, I want to consider critically whether a separation of these forms of activism from each other, based on the tasks they engage in, is legitimate. I argue that, despite their visible differences, all are principally underpinned by a commitment to addressing inaccessibility.

Throughout I want to frame addressing inaccessibility as a distinctly political contribution. To explain this point, I consider the difference between work to establish abortion pathways – a framework increasingly discussed and applied in abortion policy research to improve access, minimize unsafe access or address interrupted abortion trajectories (Coast et al., 2018) – with abortion trail activist work relating to access. Drawing from the work of Sara Ahmed on phenomenological diversity work (Ahmed, 2020), I contend that abortion trail activism practices accessibility work as a means to develop a fuller understanding of and knowledge regarding the lived barriers to abortion and work through these from a range of positions, the knowledge generation process in a continuous project of learning what Ahmed depicts as the shifting, but persistent, walls embedded within institutional contexts. This is different from abortion pathway work which tries to improve accessibility with the assumption that it is possible to definitively address barriers.

A shared activism

The four accounts of abortion trail activism outlined in the Introduction could be, if one wished, read as describing discrete forms of health activism which deal with a similar topic (abortion) but are inherently different. Viewed collectively, the excerpts from interviews and ephemera could easily be separated into two types of activism, one that involves practical work which supports abortion travellers and one which does not. Groups like LASS and the Netherlands-based group offer support that addresses the challenges presented by having to travel (accommodation, excess costs, the logistics of out-of-country travel). Mobilizations working inside national borders, trying to provide practical support at a local level, do not offer this support. Nor, indeed, do they necessarily see support to travel to clinics as a positive step. The Socorristas argue that such strategies, adopted uncritically, reinforce systems of reproductive control, albeit biomedical ones. Equally, we could separate the four accounts into 'activism that provides information', 'activism that provides hosting' and 'activism that provides financial support'.

However, treating the organizations referenced earlier as entirely different requires both the use of some very blunt instruments to guide our definitions and an acceptance to ignore that activism responds to context. For example, if we use travel, we agree to derive our understanding mainly from *who* the groups were or are supporting rather than from the issues they were/are responding to, LASS becomes defined as an Irish abortion travel movement, ignoring the fact that it was not based in Ireland and did not travel. Focusing on travel is also somewhat misplaced as the core interest of both LASS and the Netherlands-based group was not necessarily making either populations or abortion technologies (such as manual vacuum aspiration or medication abortion) more or less mobile but addressing mobility *inequality* (Hidayati, Tan and Yamu, 2021). The challenges that directed both LASS and the Netherlands-based group were disadvantages in access – they identified a political situation whereby some individuals or communities were/are either less able to access care or accrued a greater burden from accessing care due to structural and systemic barriers. Similarly, separating the groups according to the tasks they perform at a particular point in time means ignoring the fact that activists' work is based on strategic decision-making within a particular context. The increased engagement in information hotlines and mapping the location of outlets where abortion pills can be found is reflective of the context within which groups like the MAMA network and *Socorristas* emerged. But these tasks do not define these groups. Their interest is reducing the barriers to abortion, barriers which, as the interviewee below notes, predominantly effects those living in a position of social disadvantage.

> I think what will happen now is that you have people who have the money, and you have people who don't have the money. If you have, it's the same old story that all the countries know, if you have the money you can fly to whichever country around that has the abortion and has doctors, because some people have the law, but you still don't have any doctors to do it, but some places they have doctors who will do it and do it well. (Abortion activist, Africa E102)

Writing in political geography, Calkin, Freeman and others (Calkin, 2019; Calkin and Freeman, 2019; Calkin, Freeman and Moore, 2022; Engle, 2022) have applied a 'mobilities' lens to understand organizations which mobilize to support abortion access in practical ways (including distributing abortion pills, providing information and financial aid) collectively. This body of research has cogently argued against separating organizations according to whether they help people to travel or not, highlighting that the advent of abortion pills and advancements in harm reduction strategies for self-managed abortion naturally resulted in the current situation where the object that moves during an abortion journey is the pill, not the person who aborts (Calkin and Freeman, 2019). Abortion trails are increasingly technological, but so is everything else.

Freeman (2020) has further presented the framework of 'abortion mobilities' – 'the movement and fixity of people and things that shape abortion access' (Freeman, 2020: 896) – as an analytic vehicle for discussing the complex array of activisms and actors collectively in relation to their effect on the embodied experience of abortion. By connecting a range of different moving and unmoving objects within the same discursive space, abortion mobilities provides a basis for a more detailed conversation about how specific sites of contestation alter the abortion experience. In particular, the architecture and modes of travel become foregrounded as having a substantial effect on abortion journeys, which Freeman discusses uses Walters' concept of viapolitics (Walters, 2015) or the role of transport in (re)constructing the embodied experience.

I agree with the principle in this body of work to look at abortion trails as composed of mobile and immobile objects and actors. Yet, the use of the terminology of 'mobilities' is challenging when the locus of analysis is abortion trail activists who, arguably, predominantly put their energies towards accessibility. While abortion mobilities is a useful analytic device for considering the individual, embodied experience of abortion, as I will argue in the remainder of this chapter, accessibility is more appropriate to considering abortion trail activism. This is more than a straightforward shift of phrasing; it requires attentiveness to the ways that abortion trail activists mediate the border between access and inaccess.

Working with accessibility reminds us that abortion trail activism is a political act intended to contest or disrupt a particular set of conditions. The risk of discussing abortion trail activism using the language of mobilities in isolation is that, for me, our analytic gaze becomes stuck on the experience of the abortion seeker. In principle, this is perfectly appropriate but it can result in a situation where we always describe activists in relation to how they interact with abortion seekers' experiences rather than critically reflecting on what political project activists are pursuing. Through accessibility, I want to encourage a greater effort towards conceptualizing the activities of abortion trail activism. This is not concepts for concepts' sake; as I will show below through theorizing the contributions of abortion trail activists, we can draw out the richness and complexity of their work. In other words, through accessibility, I want to reinforce the presence of abortion trail activists as *activists* who are trying to fundamentally alter the terrain in which abortion exists through strategic actions rather than *actors* who soothe the sharper edges of coerced and unjust abortion (im)mobilities for individuals through practical support.

A further contribution of accessibility is that it pays attention to the precision of the work of abortion trail activists. Abortion trail activism does not address or contest all factors shaping abortion journeys equally. Their work is often, as in the organizations already mentioned, limited to information hotlines or arranging transport from ports to clinics. At face value, one could read this as proof of the limited role of abortion trail activism in the overall project of expanding abortion access. However, if we apply an accessibility approach, it is also possible to read the targeting of activist energies at certain tasks as demonstrative of meticulous strategic decision-making on their part.

Additionally, examining abortion trail activism as 'accessibility politics' opens up space for an important discussion, which I will return to later in this book, on the collaborative relationship between abortion trail activism and health services and how recognition of such collaborations challenges a framing of abortion trails as existing in the shadows. The work of abortion trail activists at different points in time and in different contexts has involved actively collaborating with health services as well as working outside them (Joffe, Weitz and Stacey, 2004). For instance, organizations such as the Liverpool Abortion Support Service connected with general practitioners involved in the Merseyside Abortion Campaign as well as health care practitioners based at the British Pregnancy Advisory Service (BPAS) to minimize fragmentation along abortion seekers' individual trail experiences. In other contexts, groups in sub-Saharan Africa work with allied health professionals – pharmacists, community health workers – to establish an abortion access network outside of urban areas.

To further substantiate my use of accessibility as a shared commitment across the diverse activist organizations previously described – and by implication a characterizing feature of abortion trail activism – the remainder of this chapter will engage with accessibility both as a general concept and as an identifiable concern of abortion trail mobilizations. My aim here is, as stated in the book's Introduction, not to rebuff the application of mobilities thinking, found in the work of Freeman, Calkin and others, as analytic approaches for understanding how abortion trail activism shapes the experience of abortion seekers. Rather it is to examine what shapes abortion trail activism as a *general* political project. In doing so, I want to move beyond describing what influences abortion trail activist mobilizing in *specific* places and at *particular* moments in time (as I did in the Introduction) towards a deeper appreciation of the underpinning concerns of *all* abortion trail activists.

At the same time, I am cautious of universalizing such a heterogeneous constellation of actors (Berro Pizzarossa and Nandagiri, 2021). It is vital that this analysis acts as a starting point for a more sustained academic conversation about abortion trail activism. Neither do I want to suggest that abortion trail activists engage with all aspects of accessibility work in the same ways, at the same time. The discussion below will note the differences in how accessibility manifests in activists' practices.

Understanding accessibility

As Ferreira and Papa (2020) discuss, mobility and accessibility differ in subtle but important ways. Mobilities considers how people move, or do not move, and under what conditions. It is about stasis and movement (Hannam, Sheller and Urry, 2006); transport and travel. Accessibility, as Ferreira and Papa (2020) write,

> is aimed at increasing the ability of people to engage with social contacts, participate in activities, and reach services; as well as increasing the ability of organisations to engage with institutional and business partners, markets, and resources. (Ferreira and Papa, 2020: 1003)

The two central distinctions between an (im)mobilities paradigm and an accessibility approach are that, first, accessibility recognizes proximity as well as mobility, advocating for a reduction in the need to move as well as improving the conditions of travel and, second, accessibility is measured through the 'effective satisfaction of needs and aspirations' as opposed to 'mobility per se' (Ferreira and Papa, 2020).

Accessibility, from this perspective, is a request by theorists and advocates to engage less with the factors and objects that render certain groups more or less mobile or what shapes the conditions and experience of travel towards addressing social and individual inequities. These inequities may be partially resolved through mobility questions – why, how and in what ways are we (im)mobile and what are the effects of this – but they are more meaningfully addressed through beginning with the understanding of what makes a contact, service, activity or experience *in*accessible.

Writing on health systems, Levesque, Harris and Russell (2013) engage with accessibility from the starting point of the individual or 'patient'. At the heart of their analysis, replicated across health literature is 'the interface of health systems and populations' (p1). These authors adopt a holistic approach to understanding access, outlining both what they see as the essential systemic 'dimensions of accessibility' –

dimensions interpreted as structural and operational characteristics – and 'corresponding abilities of populations' necessary 'to generate access'. The question here, similar to that asked by Ferriera and Papa, is what enables or limits individuals to move from the 'outside' of systems or services that they need to the 'inside'.

Dimensions of accessibility	Population abilities
Approachability	Ability to perceive
Acceptability	Ability to seek
Availability and accommodation	Ability to reach
Affordability	Ability to pay
Appropriateness	Ability to engage

Levesque, Harris and Russell (2013).

Levesque et al. locate their model of accessibility within the broad field of public health where access discussions have focused on the 'point of entry' into safe health systems. This point of entry orientation is heavily influenced by writing of health economists and public/population health analysts based in the United States and the United Kingdom since the 1970s. Interventions such as Salkever's paper 'Accessibility and the Demand for Preventative Care' interrogated and proposed solutions to the 'entry point' problem. Although there has obviously been substantial expansion and diversification of this discussion, both in terms of the geographic scope of research and the sector of the health system centred by researchers, the early arguments of Salkever and others has still substantial influence over how access is understood by health academics and policy stakeholders. Their work presented the access problem as a debate about the *utilization* of health care services and how this could be ensured by the state. While, as Levesque et al. note, there is continued disagreement over whether the interventions should focus on the characteristics of health providers, the process of care, the broader ecology of health provision or the circumstances of populations, the fact that access is about ensuring utilization/entry through a combination of health system alterations and population-level interventions has not changed.

But what makes a service, if we are to maintain the analytic object of health research, less accessible to some? This was a directing question of Ribot and Peluso's (2003) *Theory of Access*, which considered access not as a right to property/things held by some and not others but rather as a description of a set of social relations or social order, whereby some people faced more barriers to deriving benefits from existing property/things than others. Taking Levesque et al.'s domains and dimensions, combined with Salkever's earlier work and Ribot and Peluso's and Ferriera and Papa's theorizations, as a guide, inaccessibility can broadly be broken down into three main types of barriers – material, epistemic and cultural. I will now look at each of these barriers in turn, highlighting how the work of abortion trail activists speaks to a commitment to addressing these.

Material barriers to access

Material barriers to accessible health span the material conditions of the individual seeking health services and the political economies and infrastructures of health. Here we drift again, at least partly, into 'mobilities thinking' as the relevant factors become things like transport arrangements and the ability to pay to get from one point to another. Abortion trail activism is characterized by assisting abortion seekers to move across these types of material boundaries. This is perhaps the actions most closely related to abortion trail activism. Work focused on travel documents at length how abortion trail activists support abortion seekers from the home to the clinic. Abortion trail activists interviewed in research for this book and elsewhere express an acute awareness of the importance of infrastructure to access. Infrastructure does not just mean institutions but the objects and processes that connect social systems (Power and Mee, 2020; Alam and Houston, 2020). Infrastructural awareness is reflected in accounts from activists in both hyper-restrictive (De Londras, 2020) and liberal abortion regimes. The quote below, from an activist in Africa, describing their organization's work exemplifies this awareness:

[organization] provides that particular service [to] young people, adolescent girls who are under eighteen [. . .] In [organization's] country, if you are under eighteen and you happen to be pregnant, legally you can have, you can terminate your pregnancy. So, [the organization] identified these young people particularly from marginalised communities and then they will accompany them to access the service, in most cases access to safe and legal, you know, most public sectors healthcare that are providing that, you know, it's a long process, accompanying, transportation.

In this description, the activist draws attention to the fact that abortion is legal in their country under specific circumstances. Regardless, access remains limited due to the lack of connection between individuals eligible for abortion access and services where abortion can be provided.

Yet applying a health access lens is instructive for appreciating that this is not the *only* access/inaccess border abortion trail activism works on. Indeed, at a global level, travel to clinics is not the main form of boundary work. Self-managed abortion using medication has been the main orientation of abortion trail activists since the late 1990s. This is precisely why an accessibility lens is useful as it reminds us that material boundaries stretch beyond physical infrastructures. From an accessibility approach, the focus is the material burdens of health care, which can be straightforward financial payments or transport but also a loss of income or the 'matter' of health (including bodily products). This is more consistent with sociological analysis of materiality. Barad (2003), famously, and other post-humanists and new materialists extend our understanding of materialities to include everything that acquires material and meaningful form. Material barriers from a health accessibility perspective are those objects and things that are so burdensome that they inhibit the use of services.

Abortion trail activists, in their accounts of the barriers to accessing abortion facing those who they support, highlight a range of material barriers as well as different steps undertaken to minimize these. This is illustrated in the quotes from interviews below:

I mean like, I'm in a lucky position at the moment, because like I'm in touch with pharmacy, like with a colleague who's a, has the pharmaceutical background and he has been able to smuggle some of the pills and this, but again, like it really relies, like I mean, it's very exclusive and limiting because it depends on women riding on private fees, for example of a friend of a friend of a friend asking, searching for those pills and then we set it up and then we, you know, like deliver, sometimes I along with other friends provide a space where people can carry out abortion if they are living with their families or they're hiding, like you know, they want it to remain in private. So, we provide this kind of a accompaniment in a very decentralized, yet not very accessible way. (Abortion activist, Africa, E104)

So, what I can say, the pills are there, in country here in town, the pills are there in the pharmacist stores, but women accessing them is not easy, why? One thing, they're very expensive [. . .] you will find that, you know, a lot of doctors, a lot of women provide that service, and if they do they will charge you probably four hundred dollars, you know, to some people they don't even have the money. At the same time, we have other service providers who can do it as, you know, for as little as five dollars. (Abortion activist, Africa, E202)

Each of these comments points to an awareness of different material burdens, ranging from having the money to pay for abortion pills or services to the proximity of outlets selling abortion pills to having access to a physical space to carry out an abortion to the burdens of hotel fees and childcare. They also point to a commitment, shared across groups transnationally, to mitigating the effects of these burdens so that people can access abortion care. This commitment largely manifests in practical work, albeit in very different forms.

Epistemic barriers to access

Accessibility debates also draw attention to the epistemic and knowledge-based barriers to care. Writing on epistemic injustice and privilege (Kidd, Medina and Pohlhaus, 2017) explores how positionalities within health encounters and health domains are stratified according to normative expectations regarding voice, authority and the legitimacy of subjects as 'knowers'. Fricker (2007) identifies two forms of epistemic injustice – testimonial and hermeneutical. The first refers to issues of silencing through framing testimonies as illegitimate. Sociological theory addresses this phenomenon in terms of issues of knowledge recognition and value. Applying Bourdieu, certain voices are devalued as they intersect with matrices of cultural and social value (Eagleton and Bourdieu, 1992). The net effect for the individual lived experience is that their perspectives and accounts are ignored or dismissed.

The second form of epistemic injustice – hermeneutical – refers to uneven political economies of knowledge and communication. The predominant concern here is disadvantage in terms of 'interpretive resources' (Fricker, 2007: 1) or the tools necessary to articulating, understanding and utilizing information and knowledge. Critical pedagogy and critical educational scholars, most obviously Friere (1996), have worked extensively on foregrounding and addressing hermeneutical injustice. Collective education praxis underlines the exclusion of particular voices and subjects as knowledge-based tools needed to engage in decision-making are unevenly distributed or provided without supporting their use.

Carel and Kidd (2014) point to epistemic privilege as a further aspect of this manifestation of inequality. From their perspective, while certain subjects are disadvantaged by testimonial and hermeneutical injustice, others are inequitably *advantaged*. This is especially the case in relation to health workers in health contexts. The ways of knowing, interpretive resources and forms of articulation of health workers accumulate more value and are treated as more valuable. Medical knowledge and the clinician voice dominates. Mignolo (2007) connects this to a colonial matrix of power which directly and explicitly privileges ways of knowing and speaking associated with Westernized science, including biomedical science.

Moving from recognition of epistemic injustices and knowledge inequalities, both social justice advocates like Friere and sociologists such as Bourdieu promote what Pot (2022) labels 'epistemic solidarity'. Friere famously identified providing individuals with the 'building blocks' for engagement as central to addressing injustices, including epistemic injustice. Bourdieu meanwhile highlighted the need to challenge the *doxa* of social relations, or the necessary forms of individual capital (including epistemic capital), required to engage meaningfully and equitably in social interactions (Eagleton and Bourdieu, 1992). Epistemic solidarity is outlined by Pot in the following definition:

> Practices of supporting others (with whom one recognises similarity in a relevant aspect) as knowers. To qualify as solidarity, these practices must involve particular costs (such as spending time, giving up privilege, or accepting risk for oneself). (Pot, 2022: 685)

The central focus of epistemic solidarity is that service using communities is actively recognized as knowers. These knowers are subjects of a discourse where the value of individual subject's knowledge is continually contested and intersects with hierarchical subject relations. Furthermore, interpretive resources are inequitably distributed; some people are better equipped to understand the information available in a way that is meaningful and adequately supports access. Epistemic solidarity in abortion access means addressing the ways through which abortion is limited by failing to adequately accept the reproductive agency of individuals or to ensure people have sufficient information to enable to exercise their reproductive agency.

Accounts from abortion trail activists point to engaging in activities that address epistemic injustice and constitute epistemic solidarity. Hermeneutic epistemic injustice and epistemic privilege are core complaints of activists as well as the centre-point of their actions. Interviewees spoke vividly about how communities seeking abortions were systemically and persistently denied equitable distribution of interpretive resources. This denial was reflected in the fact that misconceptions about abortion continued to circulate. As the following activist, based in Africa explains:

Information about safe methods almost never existed. People always believed that having an abortion will be risking your life and that continues to sort of be the belief even now, to sort of believe that you would be risking your life but it's better to risk your life if you still don't want to get pregnant. So, just take your chances, if you survive you survive, if you don't that's probably okay as well. And we wanted to change that narrative that no, it doesn't have to be. (Abortion activist, Africa)

It is important to unpack such quotes to understand fully and recognize 'interpretive' hermeneutic epistemic (in)justice work. The first and final sentences are instructive. Both point to the fact that abortion trail activism is not just about providing information in neatly packaged data objects. It is about disrupting, through direct repackaging of information, education work and communication work the established knowledge environments that obscure the pathways to access.

The problem, from a health care access perspective, is not the absence of informational objects. Informational landscapes are saturated by data. The problem is that saturation results in entropy – all health seekers hear is noise. The people most negatively impacted are the people disadvantaged in other ways (Whitelaw, 2008). They do not have, are not provided with and/or are not supported in using tools which reduces noise. Returning to the activist's comments above, abortion trail activists' work is not directed at injecting information but addressing noise and ensuring that the messages that are conveyed do not limit the reproductive autonomy of individuals. They intervene in a space where knowledge of abortion frequently circulates – people know about it, there is information available to them – but communications do not support people to access abortion in ways that are safe or empowering. The injustice is epistemic. The access/inaccess border is not the product of information absence, it is the product of what and how information is communicated.

Again, there are several points that demonstrate that the knowledge and information work of abortion trail activists is not just about injecting information but about disrupting the epistemic political modalities that limit abortion access. First, there is the comment about addressing assumptions about payment and cost. Again, this is not about an absence of information but the circulation of inaccurate communications coupled with a lack of interpretive skills necessary to exercise or take advantage of health rights and entitlements. The result is inaccess. As the activist working in the Netherlands quoted at the beginning of the Introduction stated, people who are entitled to a free abortion will not access it because the law is obscure. Second, and again this indicates that the work of abortion trail activists is about addressing epistemic hierarchies, this activist noted that the inaccurate information is communicated by clinic staff. Approached through the epistemic injustice framework, the status of health facility workers as dominant 'knowers' enables them to make abortion inaccessible even though the information they communicate is factually incorrect.

The accounts from research participants also illustrate how abortion trail activisms take on the burden for addressing epistemic injustice. Social movement researchers such as Pot (2022) address this as *epistemic solidarity*. Accounts from activists in historic and contemporary trail activist groups indicate that, while epistemic solidarity translates into a diverse range of specific activities, treated collectively it reflects a shared awareness of and committed to addressing epistemic injustice. Among specific actions, abortion trail activists described establishing infrastructures for addressing misunderstandings about abortion as well as distributing information that clarifies and signposts pathways to abortion care. These actions, as the quote below from a former member of the Liverpool-based group ESCORT describes, were often directed at individual abortion seekers:

> We would talk a bit on the phone to the person and make sure [. . .] they had access to information before they came. Practical information they may not have through of before coming over. (ESCORT 1).

It is crucial to recognize that, as already stated, there is more work going on here than simply providing information. This interviewee described, during our conversation, a comprehensive programme of support aimed to address the factors, related to information and understanding, which could inhibit access to abortion. These ranged from directions from airports or ferry terminals to abortion clinics, to requirements about waiting times and fasting expectations. Abortion trail activists interviewed in the research for this book were attentive, and keen to stress that addressing epistemic barriers to access is not solely achieved through distributing contact details of abortion providers. As the comment from an African activist below indicates, trail work involved supporting women develop the interpretive tools to feel comfortable and confidant to access abortion (in this case through self-managed abortion):

> as much as we're talking about self-medical abortion, it's not just an easy thing for women to do, and the reason why I'm saying it's not just an easy thing is because women have that fear of if the pills are going to be successful because they've heard of other women dying because of going for an abortion. Like women are still stuck into this is abortion safe or unsafe? So, for the ones that at least land into our hands, or for the ones that are able to attend some of our sessions, they're able to know that we have safe abortion, that a woman can have below the twelve weeks very safely and there is a place she can access the pills and even use them at home without involving any doctor.

But epistemic solidarity is demonstrated in other ways. In hyper-restrictive contexts where information sharing and communications between health information 'knowers' and abortion seekers are the specific targets of anti-abortion law and policy, it can also involve absorbing the burden of developing strategies to work around the law. Later in their interview, the activist quoted above explained their work involves both supporting abortion seekers developing necessary interpretive skills to access abortion pills and protecting pharmacists who stock abortion pills from the pharmacy poison boards who restrict access to these medicines:

> the stigma that surrounds the whole process, so you'll find most of the women we see are not been known that she has used the pills,

providers also don't want to be known that they're the ones who are making the pills accessible to these women and girls, because of the stigma. Labelling of names, they're going to be labelled names, and that is why most of them will do it, but they want to do it secretly. But for the providers that we train, we look for pharmacists that are registered, and they're allowed legally to stock the pills, and these are the pharmacist stores that you find now the other small retailers will go to them and buy their pills from them. So, there is one thing that the pharmacists told us, that sometimes it's a challenge to them when women are coming to access these pills, so they always have a book of record where they record the number of pills that they have sold in the stock. But now when the pharmacy poison boards come it really inspects on that, to know who bought this pill? They're supposed to sell to their retailers, not through, like through another chemist that is coming to buy the pills to go and go sell to PPH, but now they're forced to start saying 'who bought this pill?', it becomes a challenge, and they cannot go on saying 'it's for a woman (a) or woman (b)', so they told us that is a very big challenge that they always go through that they have their own ways on how they manage on their records, that we don't go in to deep, we don't ask them 'how do you do it?', because our purpose is women accessing those pills and using them safely.

It also involved, as the quote below indicates, ensuring that, when an abortion seeker reached a doctor they were trained and knew how to perform an abortion.

really the access to services for abortion, it's too dependent on the will of people to risk some hard times, you know. And the problem is that generally speaking we don't have a lot of doctors when it comes to gynaecology and surgical expertise in that field, so even if you find somebody who accepts there's no guarantee that that person knows what they are doing.

Abortion trail activists are keenly aware of these factors. Their efforts to reduce the border between access and inaccess partly involves shifting the responsibility to communicate abortion information away from health professionals who may put themselves at risk. This includes information about where and how to access abortion in a way that respects the decision-making and autonomy of individual abortion seekers. Globally there is a range of different manifestations of how abortion trail activists protect or take the information-provider responsibility away from health professionals. Information hotlines, such as the Women's Information Network in Ireland in the 1980s and 1990s and contemporary Safe2Choose network (which has a global reach) and Argentinian Lesbians and Feminists for Abortion Rights network, exemplify this form of epistemic solidarity. In each of these instances, activists strengthen understanding and awareness of where to access abortion through clearly and directly communicating with abortion seekers.

There is a distinction that needs to be drawn here between distributing information – which may not resolve inaccess if interpretive and heuristic gaps remain unaddressed – and providing information to facilitate access. It is this distinction that a health access perspective underscores. While abortion trail activists do both, their primary objective is to address interpretive gaps and epistemic disadvantage. Organizations such as Safe2Choose have created multiple platforms including the webchat facility mentioned in the quote above. Other groups such as the Socorristas in Red and the Red Compañera have produced 'hotmaps' of reliable providers. In Africa, hotlines like Aunt Rosy (Nigeria) and Aunty Jane (Kenya) maintain webchat and telephone hotlines. The commitment to providing information to facilitate access is reflected in the quotation below from a member of Safe2Choose,

> Safe2choose, lo que hace es brindar un asesoramiento general sobre temas de aborto, tenemos consultoras . . . bueno más que consultoras son consejeras en realidad, sería la traducción exacta. Ellas son las personas con las que . . . si vos necesitás realizar un aborto y llegas a nuestras páginas, ellas son las personas que te van a asesorar. Hay un chat ahí donde puedes hablar con ellas. Te van a brindar la información pertinente.

> Safe2choose, provides general advice on abortion issues, we have consultants ... well, more than consultants, counsellors would be the exact translation. They are the people with whom ... if you need to perform an abortion and you come to our pages, they are the people who will advise you. There is a chat there where you can talk to them. They will provide you with the pertinent information.

This interviewee's use of the term *'pertinente'* is significant here, as is their description of their information service as a dynamic exchange or dialogue with abortion seekers. Once again, the role of abortion trail activism is not disseminating information into a void – although at an earlier point in the discussion, this particular interviewee agrees that some jurisdictions are devoid of access support – but addressing a series of epistemic challenges. Abortion seekers are knowers of their own reproductive health wishes but lack the interpretive tools to identify or use effective abortion methods; interpretive tools are intentionally targeted and disrupted; and health professionals' ability to engage in knowledge sharing is frequently constrained. Abortion trail activism is not advertisement; people know abortion exists. It is epistemic solidarity.

An image of abortion trail activism as epistemic solidarity is further supported by the fact that the information work of activists is burdensome and involves close working with individuals and communities who are less able to 'read' or use the information technologies required to access abortion. These include consent forms and bureaucratic, administrative documents.

> So through that, they identify these different young girls and they work with the families to identify are the families willing to go ahead and consent or provide guidance or authorisation that these children can actually, actually they are children yes, and what they can really provide to get that service. So, you will find that you know, those who are already identified are already from poor backgrounds, those who probably didn't complete school, whose parents don't have any income, and so what they do is they really accompany them from wherever

they are to the health centre and they're able to connect them with the health centres, as you know find all the papers.

As this interviewee's account illustrates, this work is complex and time-consuming. These actions do not come without personal risk. The work of clearly communicating where to access an abortion within contexts where, as in Ireland and parts of Africa and Latin America, the borders between access and inaccess are entrenched through reprisals against information sharing lies at the peripheries of illegality. Interviewees working with information hotlines who participated in the research for this book described personal repercussions for activists, including police raids and arrests. Interviewees from abortion trail activism also highlighted the emotional burden of addressing epistemic barriers. Indeed, activists supporting abortion seekers in multiple jurisdictions described the emotional labour as one of the most challenging aspects of activists' work.

These activists emphasized the difficulty of sustaining their organization without their members, the majority of whom participated on a voluntary basis, becoming burnt out. Indeed, even for those organizations who had full-time members, the complexity of navigating epistemic borders and toll of curating the information needs to ensure someone who was able to access an abortion was intensely emotional. It involves, as the interviewee below, working in the United States notes, becoming deeply familiar with the personal life circumstances of the abortion seeker and work closely with them during a period of heightened emotional stress:

> From the co-ordinators perspective, this is work that can be very emotionally taxing for people. There is a high volume; there is a lot, wide range of emotions that people are experiencing in that moment. Especially when they have to leave their homes for days at a time. There is – you know and that's not even bringing into it the stigma that our clients are experiencing and how that can get transferred onto co-ordinators and even if and when you are able to identify other resources and referrals to provide emotional support – you as a human

doing this work will inevitably feel that and experience that. So just from a co-ordinator perspective this work is profound and emotionally layered. (TN102)

Cultural barriers to access

The third barrier foregrounded by adopting an accessibility lens is cultural. For abortion this mainly involves stigma and the existence of a transparent conversation about where and how to access abortion. To illustrate this barrier, some interviewees drew on their own experiences with abortion. In her interview, a *parcera* activist in Colombia compared two personal abortion experiences. The first time she had an abortion, during her teens, was an isolated and isolating experience. Still living with her parents and attending school, the interviewee found the abortion traumatic and stigmatizing. She was unsure where to access abortion and ended up using an unsafe provider. The second time she sought an abortion was vastly different. This time, she attending university and she was supported by friends. She was recommended where to go to access an abortion and encountered incomparable levels of care, including the support of a *parcera*.

While both abortions occurred in the context of limited abortion access, both this interviewee's abortions took place before the expansion of legal abortion in Colombia under a 2006 Constitutional Court ruling, in her account the interviewee presented two entirely different experiences of accessing abortion. It was after her second abortion, she explained, that she fully realized the violence of anti-abortion environments. Her first abortion was traumatic not just because of legal restrictions or even the attitudes of the people around her. It was the isolation and need to self-navigate without any information as to where or how to access abortion in Colombia.

Cultural barriers and stigma impact the circulation of information about how and where to access abortion. They also affect the treatment of abortion within health services themselves, with access limited by misconceptions about the permissibility of abortion care on the part of medics, state institutions and the publics. As the Kenyan case detailed in the Introduction showed, even where there are legal pathways to abortion, health care providers who offer abortion services and abortion seekers can experience retribution by the criminal justice system. This is rooted, according to activists, in a stigmatizing attitude that abortion is not a legitimate, or indeed legal, form of health care. The cultural framing of abortion as problematic, as described by the African activist quoted below notes, is separate from the desires and needs of the population, for whom abortion is a wanted and essential form of health care:

> There's still a lot of stigma around abortion because even with the most liberal people, people still will treat people who are seeking abortion very differently. But yes, people just, this is the funny part, the funniest part about abortion is that you find someone who was against us two years ago and saying we were going to hell because we were pushing for women to make their own choices would be the ones coming two years later asking for information where to get safe abortions because they either got pregnant, their daughter got pregnant, their girlfriend got pregnant, you know people need you when now it's their turn.

Stigma or stigmatizing attitudes act here as an accessibility barrier. They constrain both health services – determining the willingness of legislators to allow them to offer abortion openly and the acceptance of abortion as an ordinary form of reproductive health care by health providers – and abortion seekers – deterring them from requesting abortion care or declaring the need for an abortion. Cultural barriers and attitudes operate affectively, as Vacarezza and Burton (2023) allude to; shaping our expectations about an abortion experience and thus allowing impediments to abortion care to persist. The silence and stigma surrounding abortion, as activists working within African communities noted, meant that there was almost an expectation that abortion would be burdensome or harmful. From an accessibility perspective, this expectation tacitly permits health systems to avoid making adjustments that would reduce the burden of accessing care.

A visible commitment across abortion trail activist mobilizations globally is challenging such expectations. This manifests in a variety of ways, ranging from radical cultural practices which celebrate abortion as an ordinary part of health care to community workshops where abortion trail activists discuss the very real ability of abortion to be both a safe and non-stigmatizing form of health care. Here, through framing abortion trail activism as committed to accessibility, we can see the shared intent behind seemingly disparate activities.

Abortion trail activism and accessibility as a political intervention

A problem with emphasizing accessibility is the temptation to reduce abortion trail activism to addressing barriers to utilizing abortion services or even informing service improvements. These concerns are articulated in recent research and writing about abortion pathways and barriers and facilitators to abortion care. Much of this literature, which is firmly located within fields of health care improvement or health service improvement, presents explanations for interrupted or unsafe abortion access and offers examples of best practice or effective resolutions. Abortion pathways research adopts a user-perspective, echoing writing on abortion mobilities, exploring barriers and facilitators along abortion seekers' pathways to care (Margo et al., 2016; Assifi et al., 2020; Srinivasan, Botfield and Mazza, 2022).

There are similarities between abortion pathways approaches and abortion trail activism. At a basic level, both emphasize accessibility as a critical problem with material, structural (i.e. availability of providers, distribution of services) and cultural components. Where the two approaches separate is at the level of praxis. Abortion pathways research generates evidence to inform service improvements, rendering abortion more accessible through addressing identifiable problematics. However, what connects abortion trail activisms is not just remedying access issues. Rather it is a shared interest in continuous reflection on persistent but shifting barriers to accessing abortion. This interest is demonstrated by the sustained work of activists in contexts where abortion legislation is more liberal, such as the Netherlands, or even where abortion has been decriminalized, such as Northern Ireland or parts of Latin America, to reach out to communities whose access needs are more complex or who may continue to face barriers to abortion. As interviewees in the projects underpinning this book explained, part of their activist work to address accessibility issues involved connecting with communities who lived at the intersections of multiple disadvantages, such as asylum seekers, sex workers or members of the trans and non-binary community.

The accessibility efforts of abortion trail activism are part of a political intervention to disrupt the boundaries between ability to use or access abortion and the inability to use/access abortion. There is a continuous component to this work, and an acceptance of incompleteness that is not emphasized as strongly in abortion pathway work, where the interest in always trying to generate and expand knowledge of the access/inaccess border is treated as less significant than identifying strategies to address accessibility. Sociological theory, particularly the work of Sara Ahmed on equality, diversity and inclusion work (Ahmed, 2012), is a useful conceptual frame here to explain the political character of abortion trail activists' efforts to address accessibility meaningfully as compared to a evidence-based policy-making approach, such as abortion pathways, where the objective is to resolve impediments.

In her main focused text on diversity – *On Being Included: Racism and Diversity in Institutional Life* (2012) – Ahmed distinguishes between non-performative diversity work and substantive, diversity work as a phenomenological practice (which I will address as *diversification*). Ahmed connects the former with problematic institutional politics of signalling but not acting on a commitment to diversity. Here Ahmed delineates between stating a commitment ('speaking diversity') and committing to act towards the requirements of that commitment. The latter requires mobilizing towards the discursive relations embedded within the diversity statement. These relations are articulated in an additional diversity language, a language of terms such as equity and inclusion.

The problem Ahmed identifies is that diversity work within neoliberal institutions – such as in academia, her object of study – frequently stops at stating a commitment or diversity talk. This is only addressed, in Ahmed's study, when 'diversity workers' (those in administrative roles focused on diversity and equity) push commitment statements into actions. However, this requires a commitment by the individuals in those roles to consistently push against institutional frameworks and cultural codes embedded and reinforced in their institutional context. In doing so, diversity workers risk becoming labelled as troublesome and facing professional reprisals and isolation as 'killjoys' (a topic Ahmed developed earlier in *The Culture Politics of Emotion* and returns to in her works *Living a Feminist Life* and *Complaint!*). Because of these governing dynamics, institutions are relatively free to claim a commitment to diversity without 'follow through' or action (Ahmed, 2012). Diversity thus becomes non-performative – it neither works (i.e. does something) nor meaningfully impacts the formation of subjects, subjectivity or discourse (i.e. acts performatively).

The ability to adopt non-performative diversity has two effects on the institutions where there are visible diversity issues (reflected in an institutional Whiteness and inequity in work trajectories). The first is that it enables institutions to claim diversity as a component of their institutional narrative. This acts as a bulwark against equity- or diversity-based criticisms as they emerge. Rather than respond and act, institutions can point to a prior statement of being committed to diversity to deflect or repudiate the criticisms. Effectively, as Ahmed outlines, institutions can respond to complaints relating to diversity (e.g. racism, gender discrimination/underrepresentation, ablism) by saying, we cannot have a diversity issue because we have already committed ourselves to diversity.

This connects to the second effect of non-performative diversity, according to Ahmed, which is the ability of institutions to present themselves as models of diversity even when they are demonstrably, and potentially visibly, not. The core of this argument is that when non-performative diversity constitutes a diversity commitment in and of itself, then the institutions engaged in non-performative diversity work can claim that they *are* emblematic of diversity even if they have taken no meaningful steps to address inequities or underrepresentation of minorities. This claim affords institutions the capacity to, on the one hand, distance themselves from accusations of diversity problems, and, on the other, obscure their lack of meaningful diversity. As a result, Ahmed argues, institutions where particular communities are clearly marginalized can continue to ignore the barriers facing these communities because the institutions *are already diverse*.

The counterpoint to this non-performative diversity work presented by Ahmed is a phenomenological practice undertaken by diversity workers. The contribution of this phenomenological practice is ultimately more meaningful and counteracts the problematic effects of non-performatively. Specifically, this meaningful diversity work limits the ability of institutions to either obscure or deny their uneven and inequitable landscapes. By phenomenology, Ahmed speaks to a theoretical orientation, drawing on Husserl's phenomenological attitude, where knowledge emerges from encounters with the norms of lived experience. In the case of diversity, Ahmed means knowledge of how institutions marginalize and limit diverse populations through the lived experience of trying to implement policies (expressed in diversity commitments) to repair and address these inequities. As Ahmed writes:

> Diversity workers acquire a critical orientation to institutions in the process of coming up against them. They become conscious of 'the brick wall,' as that which keeps its place even when an official commitment to diversity has been given. Only the practical labour of 'coming up against' the institution *allows this wall to become apparent*. To those who do not come up against it, the wall does not appear – the institution is lived and experienced as being open, committed, and diverse. (Ahmed, 2012: 174, emphasis in original)

The 'doing' component of Ahmed's more meaningful form of diversity work is critically important to her account of how diversity work can be made meaningful. In addition to allowing the wall to become apparent, diversity workers can draw forth new understandings of contours of the wall and, importantly, 'what does or does not get across' (Ahmed, 2012: 175). Significantly, from her research with diversity workers, Ahmed contends that their contribution to projects of equity and social justice lies in continuing to highlight and make apparent the persistence of 'brick walls' in institutions who have already laid claim to the achievement of diversity. Approached as a phenomenological practice, diversity work 'is a refusal to look away from what has already been looked over' (Ahmed, 2012: 183).

As Sara Ahmed (2012) argues, diversity without meaningful disruption of discursive relationalities or subjectivities (diversification) can work to protect organizations from criticism related to or critical reflection on internal hierarchies and inequalities. Focusing on diversity work in Higher Education Institutions, Ahmed contends that the language of diversity can be used as public relations and 'be mobilized in defence of an organization and its reputation' (Ahmed, 2012: 144). Continuing this line of argument, Ahmed proposes that diversity language can be mobilized to limit the inclusion of those voices and bodies which do not fit within a taxonomy of 'acceptable difference'. This is expressed in the quote below:

> The discourse of diversity is one of respectable differences – those forms of differences that can be incorporated into the national body. Diversity can thus be used not only to displace attention from material inequalities but also to aestheticize equality, such that only those who have the right kind of body can participate in its appeal. (Ahmed, 2012: 151)

The distinction Ahmed raises is between a presentation of diversity by organizations or corporate entities – including large movements cutting across numerous actors – on the basis of the heterogeneity of their membership and an active commitment to diversifying discourse through disrupting power relations, engaging with other histories and voices and challenging dominant norms.

Returning to accessibility and abortion trail activism, Ahmed's provocations on diversity work suggests that there is a meaningful difference between, on the one hand, a commitment to developing critical consciousness of barriers experienced by those in discursive positions of disadvantage and exclusion and translating that knowledge into practices to address such barriers and, on the other, an exercise in resolving issues of exclusion or definitively remedying barriers. The former is a political praxis, where knowledge and activism are continually expanding understanding about access/inaccess borders, who they apply to and under what conditions. This is an activism that is continually remaking and revising abortion trails and abortion trail activism. The latter is a more functionally and problem-oriented project which, while important for addressing inequities, can become fixed in time if evidence is organized in support of a specific accessible framework. The room for exercising a phenomenological attitude is lost in a context of designing a pathway whereas the effervescence of trails affords space for change.

Conclusion

This chapter has tried to further excavate the depth and complexity of activism that, at face value, seems to be principally a 'doing'. While abortion trail activism manifests in practical actions, these actions are underpinned by and part of a distinct political project. At the core of this project, this chapter argues, is a commitment to addressing and minimizing the barriers between access and inaccess. The chapter has drawn attention to three barriers to access that abortion trail activisms work to address – material, epistemic and cultural. Again, while the image of abortion trail activism is admittedly partial, the chapter provides a means of recognizing and discussing abortion trail activism beyond an identity defined by function. Using Ahmed's arguments on meaningful diversity work as a guide, the chapter also highlighted the resolutely political character of abortion trail activism as opposed to work on constructing more accessible abortion pathways. Later in this book, I will return to this point to consider the contestations within pro-choice abortion politics between pursuing formalization of abortion trails under the auspices of a State-sanctioned abortion care architecture and amplifying the positive aspects of abortion trails.

2

Care

Introduction

The preceding chapter illustrates both the possibility of connecting the disparate activist movements that circulate within and work on the informal, unsanctioned and collective networks facilitating abortion as orientated towards and manifestations of a shared political praxis. Recognizing the cross-jurisdictional diversity and nebulousness I proposed an equally nebulous term – abortion trail activism. In Chapter 1, I contended that a characteristic of abortion trail activism is its concern with accessibility. Importantly, I argued that abortion trail activisms demonstrate a political interpretation of accessibility work rather than solely a functional or solution-focused approach.

To explain this point, I drew on Ahmed's conceptual interventions on phenomenological diversity work as a praxis of generating knowledge and understanding of complex and lived barriers. Ahmed counterpoints this with diversity work aimed to concretely identify and address inclusion solutions, which she indicates are underpinned by a neoliberal, managerial logic. This neoliberal diversity work, Ahmed's writing implies, is often a process of foreclosure, where manageable problems are emphasized over complex, persistent and emergent challenges.

Abortion trail activism, like Ahmed's phenomenological diversity work, is characterized by an enacted interest and concern with drawing attention to more complex barriers to access. These can only be recognized when the experiences of those who encounter such barriers are engaged with. The difference is an effort, which is resolutely a political intent, to continuously reach out and generate new knowledge about those who need and use abortion trails. Although the context and form of abortion trail activist groupings globally are diverse, this commitment, I argued, is a shared one.

This chapter will develop further the argument that the various groups who work on abortion trails are reflective of a commitment to practising a feminist ethic of care. As part of this discussion, the chapter will consider the presence of Aunts on abortion trails as indicative of abortion trail activists' engagement with care as political praxis. It will then outline what a feminist ethic of care means and outline how this is practised through activist work in different jurisdictions.

On Aunties

One of the most fascinating points on my own trail through the landscape of abortion activism occurred when I realized I was surrounded by aunties and female kin (familial and non-familial). I had been aware of the use of 'visiting an aunt' or referencing aunts or female relations who 'went abroad' as an established colloquial euphemism for gendered health migration (including, but not only, for abortion services) in Ireland. The association of travelling to aunts, travelling aunts, mysterious female relatives and female family friends living in England is woven so tightly into cultural narratives and histories of Ireland, pregnancy and abortion that, in the opening scenes of the hit TV show *Derry Girls*, Danielle introduces her cousin James as the (previously unknown) child of her 'aunt who went to England for an abortion but didn't get one' (*Derry Girls*, season 1, episode 1). Similarly, Eva O'Connor's 2015 play *My Name is Saoirse*, set in 1980s Ireland when abortion was legally restricted, in which the protagonist finds herself pregnant, explicitly connects abortion access and visiting an aunt living in England (O'Malley, 2019) through the advice Saoirse receives from her more worldly friend Siobhán about how she can access abortion:

My grandaunt Rita lives over there. She's a fierce nice woman. She helped my cousin a few years' back, she was in a much worse position than you are now. Sure Rita's lonely over there. She'd love to have a few visitors. I'll give her a ring, see what she can do for us. (O'Connor, 2015: 21)

I also already knew that organizations in the United States and Ireland in the 1970s and 1980s, supporting access to abortion when the procedure was criminalized, would advise abortion seekers to use set women's names or say they were calling a friend rather than name the organization. The Jane Collective is probably the most well-known example of this tactic but the London-based Irish Women's Abortion Support Group (IWASG) also occasionally operated under the name Imelda (Rossiter, 2009). However, Jane and Imelda were not aunts and were used as security measures. By speaking to Jane or Imelda, the abortion seeker could continue to conceal their pregnancy and individual activists did not have to reveal any personal identifying details. Identification, in both the US *pre-Roe vs Wade* and Ireland in the 1980s and up to the 1990s, was an active concern. Provision of abortion support was a criminal offence. Secrecy was paramount. Other movements in Ireland, such as the Women's Information Network (WIN), also tried to hide individual members' identity. One former member, who I interviewed in August 2020, said that they still did not know everyone who was involved.

Even with this prior knowledge, I was not expecting aunts to feature so prominently in the current abortion landscape. But aunts are still everywhere. Abortion seekers are still encouraged to call Aunt Barbara (Poland), Aunty Jane (Kenya, Uganda) and Aunt Rosy (Nigeria, Malawi). My first reaction to these new-found (to me) aunts was that, like Imelda and Jane, they were a way for activists to remain anonymous and for abortion seekers to receive support in confidence. I thought they may also serve a similar narrative purpose to Danielle's aunt and James' mother in *Derry Girls* – a woman who had travelled because she was pregnant, out of wedlock and culturally out of place – or Siobhán's grandaunt Rita in *My Name is Saoirse* – a lonely woman who offers emotional support and accommodation for abortion travellers. These readings arguably reflect my own location within and familiarity with the established discourse of abortion trails. Aunts on the trails, in the Irish/US context, are there to hide abortion, offer informal emotional or logistical support, or warn against it.

Certainly, there were similarities, most obviously reflected in the association of 'going to see an aunt' and receiving reproductive advice or support. The African Abortion Aunts, for example, act as waymarkers on trails for abortion and other forms of sexual and reproductive health care guidance or advice. However, at a deeper level, Aunty Jane is a challenge to Jane's colonization of abortion histories, where women's names are signifiers of solidarity or a concealment tactic. While a hotline allows volunteers to remain anonymous, it is not used solely for security purposes. Aunty is used to encourage access and advertise services. Women's names as mechanisms for hiding abortion is a Global North history. In the Global South, women's names are also strategic devices for speaking openly about abortion in the public sphere. This difference is more acutely reflected in the fact that, while Jane answered the phone, Aunty Jane speaks out and amplifies accurate information about how and where to access abortion services through social media. Aunty Jane has her own hashtag – #BongaAuntyJane – encouraging people seeking advice on all aspects of reproductive health, bodily autonomy and intimacy to use the service. The Janes may have been activists, but they were never as active as Aunty Jane is. Aunty Jane intervenes into public silences, and silencing, of reproductive conversations.

Activist abortion Aunts are not a prominent feature of academic literature on abortion access. This absence is in itself an oddity, given how strongly aunts and aunting features within debates about sexuality, gender and reproductive governance. In Margaret Atwood's novel *The Handmaid's Tale*, the subsequent hit TV show, and the original novel's companion piece, *The Testaments*, Aunts and aunting are central to the hyper-restrictive reproductive governance system in Gilead. While Gilead is imagined as an ultra-patriarchal society, with an active male militia, the Eyes, the Aunts have the most direct control over reproduction. They act as wardens of Handmaids, monitoring their adherence to systems of reproductive control and both orchestrating and doling out punishments for rule-breakers.

Outside of Atwood's very specific use of the label aunt in White, Global North fiction, aunts are hugely significant figures in Global South cultures. This significance has not gone unrecognized by artists and writers or, more recently, by scholars. South Asian Studies now contains a burgeoning academic conversation about 'Auntyness' and the Aunty. The figure of the disciplinary/reproductive governing aunt is found in cultural representations of Aunties in Asian literature and filmography. As the Asian-American author, Maria Qamar, in the introduction to her 2017 book *Trust No Aunty* notes:

> Aunty is a term of endearment (and sometimes insult) used to describe an older woman. The aunty is a cross-cultural phenomenon that isn't limited to a family member; she could be a neighbour, a family friend, or just some lady on the bus who wants to throw some casual black magic your way. Most commonly featured in Indian soap operas, an aunty is a feisty and dramatic powerhouse of a woman who enters your house with plans to take over your life for a very small and strangely particular reason. When aunties combine into groups of two or more, their plotting power is instantly multiplied. They are at family parties or friendly get-togethers with your mother, finding ways to make your life difficult, trying to get you married to their sons, and telling you to lose weight while simultaneously trying to feed you a second dinner. (Maria Qamar, 2017: 1)

Qamar's presentation of the Aunty echoes the dominant framing of Asian Aunties, or more specifically Indian Aunties, in popular culture and cultural studies. Khubchandani (2022) documents how Bollywood filmography includes numerous examples of Aunties who actively engage in surveillance and 'police gender and sexual freedoms' (Khubchandani, 2022: 2).

That said, Khubchandani, and the nascent field of 'critical aunty studies', challenges the simplistic framing of Aunties as reproductive governors. While the Aunty is frequently visually and narratively positioned on the margins in cultural representations – in the TV adaptation of *Handmaid's Tale*, the first dedicated episode to an Aunty does not occur until mid-way through the show's third season – they occupy a *liminal* rather than a *marginal* discursive subject-position. This distinction is critical. Liminality is ambivalent and complex, it is a between space whose subjects move across discursive terrains. A liminal subjectivity is more agile and can combine multiple components. As Khubchandani outlines:

> The term 'aunty' bursts with meanings that exceed its naming of a social relation, offering more and messier ways to interpret gender and kinship. Aunty works differently from friend, sister, mother, women, lady, or person and disorganizes normative social relations: aunty 'return[s] names to women who [have] been lost to marriage and children. . . . Instead of "wife to" or "mother of," women could be Auntie Jane or Auntie Mary."' (Khubchandani, 2022: 2)

Working through queer theory and porn and drag representations, Khubchandani presents an imagine of the Aunty as an agile, playful, femme identity which defies a single, cis-gendered/heteronormative female subjectivity. Again, there are cultural examples of this queer or queering Aunty. The Auntie in Aditi Brennan Kapil's 2013 plan 'Braham/i' 'filters pornography, sex education, and anti-colonial history into her sibling's home, offering an intersex kid illicit knowledge with which to think and make their gender' (Khubchandani, 2022: 354). Meanwhile, in the 1990s British-Asian comedy sketch show *Goodness Gracious Me* and its spin-off chat show *All Round to the Kumars*, the Aunty figures are the most obviously subversive in terms of their engagement with heteronormative subjectivities and discourses. Even where they are played as socially conservative, the Aunties in *GGM* and *Kumars* disrupt norms through articulating conservative ideals to absurdity and excess. The subversive, sexualized Aunty is also presented in *Derry Girls* through the character of Aunt Deirdre – who went to England for an abortion but did not get one – who returns briefly in season two as a largely disruptive, irresponsible and sexually active counterpoint to the other older female characters.

In their discussion of aunting practices and relationships, Ellingson and Sotirin (2006) suggest that 'aunting schemas are likely to reflect other culturally significant female figures' (p487), drawing reference to US-based Black feminist writing on 'othermothers' (Collins, 2005) and the importance of the 'godmother' in BIPOC kinship. Aunties here are akin to shared matriarchs but not necessarily connected to maternal identities or bonds. In the Global North and South, there are again clear representations of the aunt-matriarch. This aunt is sometimes represented as explicitly not a mother, like the Irish author Frank McCourt's aunts in his autobiographical work *Angela's Ashes*. All of McCourt's aunts were childless, and none of them could be described as empathetic or 'caring', but throughout his account they are all identified as providing essential financial and practical support.

The matriarchal aunt is a shared feature of Global South societies. Again, in the Asian context, as Tincknell (2020) describes:

> The terms 'Auntie' and 'Uncle' are widely used within sub-continent and diasporic Asian cultures as generic honorifics to describe middle-aged or older non-family members as well as those in the extended family. Every older female is 'Auntie' even when she is only remotely related to the speaker. The Asian Auntie is, then, a universal figure, omnipresent in extended family networks and quasi-familial relations. Aunties are both benign and potentially dangerous, subject to mockery and condescension but also respected and feared by younger people. They dispense advice, spread gossip, proffer wisdom, and endear and annoy in equal measure. Described by the NDTV website devoted to Indian popular culture as 'omnipotent and omnipresent', Aunties can be frumpy, grumpy and repressive or liberating and liberal. (Tincknell, 2020: 136–7)

The use of Aunty as an honorific for those who dispense advice and wisdom resonates with the use of the term Aunty in Maori culture. For the Maori, Aunties or Auntys are community elders who protect and maintain indigenous histories and knowledges, particularly those related to health and well-being. So significant is this role, that population health programmes in New Zealand have recently, and successfully, worked with and through Aunty networks and community relationships to improve Maori health.

'African Aunties', insofar any subjecthood within the African space can be generalized (see, Dosekun, 2021, for critical analysis), contain traces of all of these Aunty subjectivities and forms of aunting. In her analysis of videos produced by women and girls from the African diaspora under the hashtag 'African Aunties' on the social media platform TikTok, Akinbola (2022) identifies three main forms of 'African Aunty' performance – deprecating, celebratory and re-staged encounters. Combined, Akinbola contends, these performance videos reflect a shared understanding of African Aunties as having 'personal and cultural importance' but enacting 'gendered surveillance, discipline and shame' (Akinbola, 2022: np). The African Aunt, echoing Ellingson and Sotirin's conceptualization of aunting, is a familiar figure but may be 'like a mentor or an intimidator' (Ellingson and Sotirin, 2006: 442).

Conceptually, Akinbola's 'African Auntie' resonates with Patricia Hill Collins' (2005) writing on race, intersectionality and the figure of the mother. Analysing US-based cultural and social imaginings of mothers, Collins argues that these do not reflect the female kinship networks within Black communities in the United States. Collins contends that key female figures who, like 'African Aunties', dispense advice and judgement, acting as mentor and intimidator, are not 'bloodmothers' but 'othermothers'. However, what is distinct about Aunties, as recent writing on Aunties in South Asian *desi* cultures by Ballakrishnen (2023), Bhardwaj (2023) and the Feminist Critical Hindu Studies Collective (2022) highlights, is that the matriarchal or mentorship role co-exists which a more ambiguous, capacious social function with regard to reproduction, gender and sexuality. Furthermore, and critically, Aunties are not mothers – blood, other or god. As such the maternal, protective relationship is not a core part of their identity or role. Additionally, unlike mothers, contact with Aunties can be inconsistent and irregular.

Reflecting on 'Aunty-care' and 'Auntyness', according to Ballakrishnen (2023), involves sitting with the juxtaposition of different 'aunty scripts' – some of which involve 'social distancing rather than intimacy' (pp. 136) and others which are more explicitly resistant to social hierarchies and order. Sitting with both as co-existent is important to Ballakrishnen (2023) as it makes one attentive to how 'aunty scripts' can be practised in subversive ways to create and nurture alternative modes of inhabiting the social world. As Ballakrishnen writes:

> Just as 'anti', when read by those who wish to see, can be a powerful tool for collaborative critique, 'aunty' could be powerful too as a similar critical tool, interchangeable with that certain definition of a generative 'anti'. (Ballakrishnen, 2023: 136)

The central point raised here is that 'Aunty care' can be a radical practice if it is pursued for this purpose. However, at different points, Ballakrishnen and others emphasize the role of Aunties in reinforcing gendered notions of respectability (Ballakrishnen writes about associating some 'auntys' with being a 'good child').

Writing on the politics of *acompañante* activism in Argentina, McReynolds-Peréz et al. (2023) distance accompaniment from familial care networks as the former is interwoven with distinct feminist political objectives that do not necessarily extend to the latter. Yet the more I reflected on the presence of Aunties in the discourse of abortion access, as well as in the list of abortion support organizations globally, the more I realized how useful 'aunting' is as an analytic device in relation to abortion trail activism and the significance of organizations adopting the figure of the Aunty. It is worth noting that abortion trail activists are not unaware of the cultural significance, particularly with regard to reproduction and gender, of the Aunty figure. As the quote from an interview with members of an activist network in Africa illustrates:

> Interviewee: Yes, so Aunty Jane is . . . uh . . . in African culture, I mean, you find that girls find it easy to . . . you know . . . there's always that aunt that you can run to and talk to, yeah?
> Interviewer: Yes

> Interviewee: Yeah, so most of the time, you find that it's not really their mother that they open up to. But if, for example, they start their period they will probably feel free to go and talk to a certain aunt. So, we thought 'why not call the hotline Aunty Jane hotline?' Because it, sort of, you know, rings a bell that this is an Aunt's phone that you can run to and they talk to you, and actually when you call it's a person that receives your call and walks with you through the journey of whatever challenge you're facing.

Like trails, Aunties are complex and, as a cultural figure, open to multiple interpretations. But why is it important to recognize and discuss the presence of aunts in relation to the political characteristics of abortion trail activism? Again, this speaks to the stated purpose of this book to discuss different manifestations of abortion support work as resonant political praxes with a long history. It also speaks to the book's aim to underline, through using the terminology of trails, that these activisms are not straightforward reactions brought into being by specific events but reflect an identifiable political commitment.

With regard to the first objective, by considering the existence of aunts in the context of abortion trail activism, it is possible to enrich our appreciation that there have always been abortion trails, that abortion trails have a long-established history and a cultural presence globally. The Aunty is a shared figure. With regard to the second objective, drawing attention to aunts in the context of abortion trail activism strengthens the argument that the work different actors engage in, while diverse, are reflective of a distinguishable political project. This requires us to take notice of the fact, as indicated for example in activist accounts of why they named a hotline Aunty, that activists engaging in interventions to support abortion access use the label Aunt or Aunty for strategic, political reasons.

We can work backwards from the existence of aunts and the strategic adoption of Aunty by activists to establish activist mobilizations in different jurisdictions, including those who do not identify themselves as 'aunts', as connected to a shared political ideology. In the proceeding chapter I centred on a commitment to accessibility as a characteristic of this ideology. Here, I wanted to highlight a feminist ethic of care. This quality is illustrated by two features of abortion trail activism: the treatment of abortion care as ontological by activists and the engagement of activists in what Corwin and Gidwani (2021) describe as 'repair and maintenance' work. As a precursor to this discussion, I wanted to provide a summary of feminist ethics of care as a political ideology which emphasizes care as non-normative and ontological and positions feminist practice as activism which addresses care inequities and uneven relations of power.

Understanding a feminist, non-normative care ontology

As a general principle, non-normative feminist framings of care seek to decouple defining care and care-fullness (Lawson, 2007) from discussions of natural morality or benevolence. Instead, this theoretical approach approaches care as a practice. This framing is underpinned by two core arguments. First, that care is an active pursuit of equitable social organization and second, that care is an intentional engagement that aims to address the material and relational problematics that reproduce uneven subject-positions between those who deliver and those who receive care. This understanding of care intentionally challenges the essential moral status of care; instead proposing that it is a matter of maintaining social life through reflection and actions. The distinction here is between a view of care as inherently reflective of benevolence or goodness and an ontological view of care as something that happens because bodies and things need it to happen. Furthermore, this conceptual consideration of care directly challenges a belief that care is innately moral through highlighting that it frequently happens in ways that are discriminatory if we do not attend to the material and discursive conditions of care. As Puig de la Bellacasa explains with regard to the first point:

> Feminist ethics of care argue that to value care is to recognize the inevitable interdependency essential to the existence of reliant

and vulnerable beings (Kittay and Feder, 2002; Engster, 2005). Interdependency is not a contract, not a moral ideal – it is a *condition*. Care is therefore concomitant to the continuation of life for many living beings in more than human entanglements – not forced upon them by a moral order, and not necessarily a rewarding obligation. (Puig de la Bellacasa, 2017: chapter 2)

The second point is centred within 'feminist ethics of care' literature associated with Joan Tronto, Bernice Fisher and others (Tronto, 1993; Tronto and Fisher, 1990; Mahon and Robinson, 2011; Robinson, 2011). This body of writing offers a schema of less-discriminatory, equitable and ultimately feminist care as a praxis which highlights and actively engages with issues of material disadvantage, diminished autonomy (of those who depend on care), embodied regulatory governance and the capacity of infrastructures facilitating care to systemically discipline subjects and deny any meaningful form of dignity, equality or justice.

Feminist perspectives of care as ontological and shaped by discourse in potentially problematic ways runs through sociological theory, particularly that focused on 'more than human' relationships and discursive analysis. The idea that interdependency is central to existence is articulated across a wide range of theoretical interventions. For instance, it underpins both Foucault's framing of subjectivity as emergent from and a contribution to discursive formation and his contentions in *Birth of the Clinic* (Foucault, 2012) that care practices and spaces are rife with technologies of government. The statement, made by Foucault in his writing on care, ethics and subjectification (Foucault, 2019), that there is no subject before discourse speaks to a perspective of interdependences as ontological; meanwhile his argument that medical practice is a manifestation of regulatory governance through which specific subjectivities and subject-positions are formed and reinforced. Science and technology studies writing on materialism and post-humanism echoes these points through the concept of *assemblages* (Deleuze and Guattari, 1988; Latour, 2007; Barad, 2007). All bodies, things, ideas and object-relations materialize and emerge from the *assemblage*; there is no *pre-assemblage* state.

From a feminist perspective, the substantial contribution of an ontological framing of care is threefold. First, it challenges a presentation of care relations as inherently normative or ethical. If care is a contingency that exists because life exists, then care relations are not, as Puig de la Bellacasa (2017) notes, innately moral or normative acts. Rather they are manifestations of how society has been organized. Again, there are clear traces of critical sociological theory here, particularly Foucault's reconceptualization of care relations (in *Birth of the Clinic* and *Madness and Civilization*) as technologies of government and control. Feminist analysis expands this point to highlight how specific norms and ideologies are woven into and conveyed through care ontologies. Notions of 'good motherhood', for example, are read into care.

According to the non-normative ontological reading of care by feminist theorists like Puig de la Bellacasa, care is ambivalent in its intent and effects and ultimately shaped by the discourse it circulates within. The existence of a relation which requires or falls into the *category* of care (e.g. abortion) does not, in itself, demonstrate a relational experience (e.g. having an abortion) which is *caring*. To avoid reinforcing problematic relations of power, a non-normative perspective contends, it is crucial to distinguish between the *existence* of care as a non-normative requisite to survival and the *operation* of care as positive or negative. If we do not distinguish the fundamental existence of care from the circulation of care-full or caring interactions, according to Murphy (2015), we risk conflating ethical care with acts which, while deeply unethical, 'feel good'. Not only this, without recognizing an ethical caring practice as resulting from active decision-making, we risk erasing the work involved in ethical caring and impact on the care giver. Writing on the 'vexation of care', Murphy highlights the fact that generalized, normative care discussions can easily enable what 'feels good' to cloud the burden of care or the potential for care to be unethical by stating:

> Projects of care, feminist and otherwise, are full of romantic temptations that disconnect acts that feel good from their geopolitical implications. (Murphy, 2015: 725)

The queer crip scholar-activists Eales and Peers (2021), emphasize the historic and persistent harms experienced by individual bodies and communities as a result of normative readings of care. In their poetic and explicitly, unapologetic querying of whether care should be reclaimed as a concept, these self-proclaimed 'Mad fat femme' and 'crip ill non-binary queerdo' (Eales and Peers, 2021: 163) write that the dominance of normative models of care underpinned by ablest and gendered logics has meant that 'care is a dirty word' (Eales and Peers, 2021). As Eales and Peers write:

> Care is a dirty word for many in our communities. 'Caregiving' has become a euphemism for often-indifferent, under-funded labor that is done to our bodies to (barely) enable our continued survival. Care is a dirty word in many of our leftist-feminist communities. Care work is a classification of highly gendered and racialized labor that remains largely unpaid, underpaid, and deeply devalued. Care is a dirty word in our Mad, disability, queer activist communities. 'Taken into care' often refers to indefinite confinement, forced extraction from communities and families, and the removal of one's right to self-determination. (Eales and Peers, 2021: 163)

In this excerpt, these scholar-activists speak to the political importance of both actively resisting and openly remembering the need to actively resist normative views of care.

The second, related contribution of an ontological framing of care for feminists is that it foregrounds how narratives of care are sites and technologies of social control and governmentality. The key point here is that the language of care has been used to entrench particular sets of – gendered – relations as 'natural'. By advocating a non-normative care ontology perspective, feminist theory directs our attention to the role of care ideologies in both enhancing and obscuring power relations and problematic subjectivities and subject positionalities. To emphasize this point, sociologists such as Phipps (2020) draw our attention to how White supremacy is obfuscated through what Tronto (2015) discusses as, at turns, 'marking' some people as more or less caring or through exploitative care relations where care work is devalued and positioned as a technical engagement necessary to do more important work. The supremacist politics of care are complex and connect with a range of feminist complaints, particularly those articulated by Black Indigenous People of Colour (BIPOC). This includes reproductive justice arguments about the hyper-surveillance of Black mothers and their historic construction as less caring towards their own children. Equally it involves the use of BIPOC women to perform care work so that White women can participate in more 'important' (and ultimately more lucrative) work. As Phipps writes:

> Supremacy is expressed in the 'care chains' through which we exploit poorer women, often migrants and women of colour, to do the labour of social reproduction while we do the more lucrative work. (Phipps, 2020: 10)

Sociology of health authors such as Murphy (2015) and feminist ethic of care scholars (Tronto and Fisher, 1990) progress political arguments relating to care and feminist critique through working from a non-normative ontological framing. Starting from an understanding of care as a condition which ideologies are read into and specific social relations enforced through, this corpus of work calls for us to interrogate and *actively* challenge the uneven positionalities and social injustices entangled with care. To paraphrase Mol (2008), what social order do we maintain through our ideas of 'good' care? More pointedly, what histories and lived presents of injustice can we shine a light on through thinking critically about the norms embedded in care? Critical disability scholars and disability advocates have consistently argued that normative orderings of care relations have limited the role of those who need care from influencing the shape and character of caring (Eales and Peers, 2021). By questioning norms woven through how we think about 'good' care we open up space to engage with the historic positioning of cared-for as passive subjects.

This brings us to the third contribution of an ontological framing of care to feminist thinking. Here the main addition of an ontological perspective is that it highlights and encourages us to interrogate norms of the subjects of and subjects who care. Such interrogation, conveyed in work on disability studies, reproductive politics, and sociologies of health, draws attention to how ideas of who deserves care, what caring relationships look like and the positionalities of carer and cared for are read into and reproduced by normative care discourses. These discourses stratify care into hierarchies of deservingness, both in terms of what needs should be cared for and who should receive care, and responsibility, in terms of who should be involved in caring relationships.

The latter is a particular problem for critical care scholars and commentators, such as the Care Collective, a collaboration between four UK-based academics, who argue in the *Care Manifesto* (2020) that normative discourses of care prioritize familial (and predominantly maternal figures) or medical personnel as the subjects most responsible for care giving. On the one hand, this allows State derogation of political responsibilities to strengthen and adequately finance infrastructures of care. On the other, it excludes those who are in a position to assist in care provision from caring relations. Applying Bourdieu, normative discourse where families/mothers or health workers are responsible for care provision establishes a specific set of interpersonal relations as the *doxa* (or requirements) of entry into care exchanges (Eagleton and Bourdieu, 1992). The *doxa* include knowledges but also, following Bourdieu, forms of human, social and cultural capital recognized as valuable and desirable by the dominant, capitalist and neoliberal social order. Subjects who do not have these valued characteristics or interpersonal relations should not and cannot provide care, even if they are willing or able to care. Adopting an ontological framing of care, scholars such as those involved in the Care Collective, propose a model of care as promiscuous. By this they mean that care relations are not predicated on the existence of specific interpersonal relations, doxa or cultural/social capital; this imagined predication is normative. Care, as a non-normative ontological interdependency, can be provided by anyone.

Positioning abortion as a non-normative care ontology and challenging the *doxa* and forms of capital read into care are consistent with the arguments of reproductive justice and reproductive governance. The demand from reproductive justice/governance to accept that abortion cannot be denied, only restricted through intersectional, uneven moral, affective and political economies speaks to a commitment to pursuing non-normative ontological abortion politics. An ontological perspective is reflected in slogans such as, 'you cannot stop abortion, you can only make it unsafe'. A non-normative ideology is demonstrated by efforts to underscore how norms are read into abortion politics, and indeed reproductive politics more broadly through the systemic denial of the ability to care to those whose knowledges and social capital have been devalued. A commitment to pursuing non-normative ontological abortion politics is shown by targeted campaigns against unequal access.

A feminist ontological politics of care, following Puig de la Bellacasa, Tronto and others, involves both an explicit recognition of care as a fundamental condition to sustaining human existence and an active commitment to protecting and maintaining mechanisms for giving and receiving care. This is expressed by Puig de la Bellacasa as involving the separation, in how we think about care, from notions of benevolence. Tronto, in her earlier writings with Fisher as well as more recent contributions to feminist care scholarship, discusses this ontological politics in terms of establishing and preserving the means to care and be cared for. What makes this a feminist project, is the intent to resist technologies of governance, particularly those rooted in social norms, economies of care and the political organization of care systems. Tronto outlines this project as involving the 'democratization' of care (Tronto, 2015) or the resistance of neoliberal policies which devalue, undervalue and underpay care work. This feminist project opens up space for pursuing non-normative modes and imaginings of care. Here I want to outline the aspects of abortion trail activism that indicate that a feminist ontological politics of care is a core aspect of their work. As a starting point, I want to discuss their efforts to establish abortion care as an ontology rather than additional or alien. I argue that this commitment is most visible in their communication work. This reflects a feminist ethics of care project of recognizing care as innate conditions of existence which are orientated and shaped by norms but not created by norms.

One of the great frustrations of activists, particularly those working in spaces where abortion is legally and socially restricted, is that abortion care has always existed. Even in contexts where, as noted in the previous chapter, activists have generated new technologies for *broadening* abortion access, they did not question the prior existence of modes of abortion care. Numerous interviewees, reflecting on their own knowledges, argued that despite attempts to restrict abortion, abortion had always been part of their communities. This complaint was articulated by the activist below, working in Africa and a member of the MAMA network:

> So in the community people don't want to hear abortion so what we do we start, we have an entry point, we start with postpartum haemorrhage, we start with several women who are giving birth, when we start with that they are ready to listen and then after we get to using the same safe abortion, abortion, so that was it. People didn't like it at times, one of our staff, somebody followed her to our office, at that time our office was in the [location], in the [location], they said 'Oh so you are the people that tell these girls to be doing prostitution?' So what is your main objective, you are working to raise the issue at school for reproductive rights, so you are the people that ask these girls to be doing prostitution. So that was the notion, but I know and to the best of my knowledge that abortion has been there before we started. I am, I will be 65 years this year, when I was small I hear that people, our elder sisters, our elder aunties some of them did abortion too and they said this one I have done abortion and this is the person that some of the elderly women helped them to do. So it has been there, if it had not been there we couldn't have had a language that covers it. (Activist, Africa, E110)

Observations such as this are a consistent theme within accounts of activists, with many arguing that they had either always been aware of abortion care. Others spoke of this awareness through recounting personal experiences. An activist who said they had been working on abortion rights in Northern Ireland for just over a decade (at time of interview), spoke of their awareness of others seeking and accessing abortion despite the restrictive legal and political environment. Another, who had participated and continues to participate in abortion trail activism in Latin America and globally, said that they remembered their mother, grandmother and neighbours meeting to support each other's abortion experience. As the activist from Africa cited above explained later in her interview:

> Yes they have ways before, because there are these elderly women that it was their job to terminate this pregnancy for these young girls and they used something like herbs. They would cook it and these girls would take the liquid inside and then they started having some I don't know if they were small contractions or what, they took it, they at times, they would grind something like spices and give to them and basically they have their own ways of doing it and they have been doing it before the English medicine came up. (Activist, Africa, E110)

Across the primary and archival data, abortion trail activists consistently committed their energies to highlighting the normalcy of both abortion care and abortion. This involved work with communities, with clinicians and medics, and with abortion seekers themselves. As the long excerpt from an interview with an African activist above indicates, among the key objectives of their activism is disrupting the notion that abortion is separate from their social histories. This is particularly important in the African context. As Chiweshe and Macleod (2018) argue, there is a persistent effort by anti-choice and anti-abortion groups to present abortion as imposed from outside. This imagined separateness was embedded in the reactions to this respondent's efforts to speak openly about reproductive decision-making, including abortion. In this instance, attempts to support abortion access were challenged as recommending schoolgirls to engage in unsafe sex work with a high risk of gender-based violence.

To address this, the respondent and her fellow activists began to speak openly about the regularity of abortion in their communities as well as the continued presence, since their own childhoods, of abortion care in the social networks they live within.

A commitment to highlighting the normalcy of abortion care is also reflected in the ephemera of abortion trail activist movements. The emotionless communication of information about where and how to access abortion, in a way that amplified and continues to amplify the existence of numerous access points for services, was inspired by an effort to disrupt the construction of abortion as an unusual form of care. Fletcher (2016) speaks about the role of abortion trail activists in 'destrangering' abortion for women travelling from Ireland to England in the 1980s and 1990s. There are numerous contemporary groups who engage in similar activities. Global online hotlines, and information providing trail activisms like Safe2Choose, established in the early 2010s, project, in both their public messaging and one-to-one exchanges with abortion seekers, an image of abortion care as an unremarkable and immutable part of what Bowlby (2012) addresses as the 'caringscape', or the 'metaphorical terrain one travels while making health decisions in one's lifetime'.

Establishing abortion care as normal and refuting the presentation of abortion as alien, strange or imported involved critically engaging with collective and individual histories. As a counterpoint to the treatment of abortion as transgressive or out of place, abortion trail activists direct their energies towards speaking about the importance of abortion and how it is and has been part of their communities' history for some time. As one activist noted, despite the institutional and political silence surrounding abortion, and the accusations they received for importing a discussion that was not part of their country's history, when they directly engaged with women they found 'women were ready to talk' (African activist, EA105).

Some activists spoke of how they also had to accept that abortion was a common and quotidian life experience. As one activist working in Africa described, they initially entered into the abortion care space believing that abortion was a taboo and innately strange, particularly to those living outside urban areas. However, through workshops with women in rural communities, they realized that almost everyone they met knew someone who had had an abortion. Abortion care was very much alive to these communities as a personal experience. Despite the stigma attached to abortion care, through these workshops, the activist was able to foreground the ordinariness of abortion as a condition of women's lives. The interviewee's realization of the normalcy of abortion is indicated in this statement:

> And I remember this group was of 15 women and 12 women had had an abortion. I remember when I did not know that abortion was that common. I, like it's something that I knew happened but just never dealt with. And being like quite shocked with, I would say, the statistic. (Activist, Africa, WA109)

These actions, engaged in different ways, at different points in time, in different jurisdictions all speak to an effort to establish abortion as ontological rather than additional. Yet challenging the narrative construction of abortion as strange or separate through collecting and sharing personal stories of abortion is not the only element of these abortion trail activists' work that resonates with writing on care as ontological. The other element involved openly connecting the importance of accepting abortion as an ordinary part of the reproductive 'caringscape' with mitigating unsafe abortion. Again, communication work, including collecting and sharing information, and personal histories are key activities that reflect the project of positioning abortion care as ontological. Often the information was based on personal experience, as in the case of an activist involved in trail activism in Latin America, who spoke of her experiences of unsafe abortion care. In other situations, the activities involved highlighting to communities and policy-makers the rates of unsafe abortion and publicly remembering those who had died due to the absence of and/or restrictions placed on provision of abortion care. An example of such remembering as a way to establish abortion care's ontological basis, that it exists and is a condition of human life, is illustrated by the story below, shared by an activist working in Africa:

> so, it was a very sad story, so in town slums and the other slums that I've mentioned we used to work with adolescent girls who are going to school and then one day we had a girl, we used to talk about access to sexual and reproductive health, but not abortion, yes, but now we had a young girl who was going to school and one day she became pregnant and she did not talk about it, but now we . . . the friends came telling us, our friend is pregnant and she tried having an abortion and this is what is happening, and then we were able to reach the girl and we took her to Hospital, but unfortunately we lost her because of the complications that she went through, and from that time, that is the time we realised that we are really . . . the girls that we are working with really need the information on access to safe abortion because if this girl could have been having this information I don't think we could have lost her, and that is the time we started now talking about abortion and within the organisation we started a hotline called Y. (Activist, Africa, E105)

This account exemplifies how speaking publicly about abortion, which this interviewee framed as a key part of their work, is used by abortion trail activists to highlight both the regularity of abortion (i.e. that it is an immutable part of human experience) and the necessity of sustaining abortion care (i.e. that preservation of human existence in the way we desire depends on support abortion care).

Practising feminist care ethics

The entanglement of experiences of care with social, political, cultural and economic structures is a central theme in Tronto's writing on feminist care ethics. As outlined in her work on democratizing care, Tronto's interpretation of feminist care ethics positions care as ontological, and thus essential to our lived experience, while concomitantly arguing that the lived experience of care is formed within and therefore shaped by discourse. Predominantly focused on the United States and Global North, Tronto bases her argument around a critique of both the impact of health economies on the quality and availability of care and the lack of care shown by state institutions towards those left behind by inadequate social security systems. A feminist ethic of care, for Tronto, involves an intentional, sustained commitment to addressing regimes which are uncaring either through negligence, neoliberal design, indifference to inequalities or a combination of all three.

Tronto's arguments emphasize the need for feminists to actively contend with the context of care and the discourse, power relations and subjecthoods it (re)produces. Attentiveness to care and a commitment to feminist care practices involves intention and action; feminists must assume a responsibility to remind us of the problematics woven through care relations and reinforced through the processes and functionings of care. Importantly, this remembering labour needs to be partnered with practical action which challenges the factors limiting care giving/receiving or rendering care giving/receiving discriminatory or restrictive. Progressing from Tronto, there has been significant scholarly attention paid to the nature of these factors, with the role of care infrastructures and subjectivities of those who require these infrastructures becoming the objects of sustained academic discussion. Feminist ethics of care needs to not just trouble, as already noted, the positioning of some forms of care as strange or alien. It needs to disrupt the infrastructures through which care is practised, accessed or delivered and recognize that these infrastructures – the material 'things' that care giving happens through and in – can be unjust or violent (Rodgers and O'Neill, 2012). It needs to disturb the formation of subjects who need these infrastructures as vulnerable, burdensome, diminished, silenced or requiring curative treatment (Albrecht, Seelman and Bury, 2001).

How does a feminist ethic of care praxis manifest in abortion trail activism? A starting point for this answer is to revisit the notion of a trail briefly. As stated in the introduction, trails are multifarious and to a degree defy a precise definition. However, a point of consensus within trail literature is that working on trails involves what Corwin and Gidwani (2021) address as 'repair and maintenance work' or the everyday work that keeps 'dwelling liveable, infrastructure working, our relationships amiable, and our planet thriving' (Corwin and Gidwani, 2021: 1). It is not insignificant that Tronto and Fisher's initial outline of a feminist ethic of care explicitly identifies maintenance work as critically important. In the context of trails, repair and maintenance work is dedicated to avert and fix breakdowns in the 'webs of material, social, economic and political interactions' (Corwin and Gidwani, 2021: 3) that we depend on in a world that is ultimately precarious and fragile. As Corwin and Gidwani write:

> Repair workers recognise this [fragility] as the reality of living with others, stemming from their material experiences working with things: things need regular attention, details matter, and nothing functions alone. (Corwin and Gidwani, 2021: 12)

Corwin and Gidwani's provocation, following Tronto and Fisher and Puig de la Bellacasa, is that repair and maintenance work, as a form of care work, is not a moral imperative or benevolent obligation but an intentional, political practice of engaging in acts which sustain our capacities to function equally. These acts are mundane, granular and dedicated to protecting the infrastructures that social functioning, specifically functioning which is care-full or caring on an equitable basis, depends on (Alam and Houston, 2020; Power, 2019; Power and Mee, 2020; Power and Williams, 2020). They are caring work on infrastructures of care. The central point within this scholarship is that infrastructures of social functioning always exist but these are frequently riven with social inequalities, fragmentation and uneven political economics. It is through mundane activities that infrastructures are imbued with the feminist ethic of care stipulated in the work of Tronto, Puig de la Bellacasa and others.

Reviewing primary and secondary data relating to abortion trails activism, the intentional maintenance and repair caring work, dedicated to supporting equitable, feminist infrastructures of care visibly flows through the work and statements of abortion trail activists. Interviewees do not start from an abstract commentary about the need for abortion care to exist somewhere or even from descriptions of how they brought infrastructures of abortion care into being; they start with accounts of their own activities and how these maintain and repair abortion trails. This repair and maintenance work results in infrastructures of abortion care which are clandestine, inaccessible and unsafe becoming more care-full and facilitative to the exercise of bodily autonomy without apology.

Let us take the example of accompaniment or *acompañante* activism. This is the most prevalent form of abortion trail activism within – and now emanating from, thanks to transnational dialogues and activist and scholarly writing – the context of Latin America and the Caribbean. To give a sense of the scale of *acompañante* activism in the region, Zurbriggen, Keefe-Oates and Gerdts (2018) have recorded 39 *acompañante* collectives operating in Argentina alone, basing this estimation on data provided by 170 activists in the country. This data does not account for the number of *acompañante* activists operating in Colombia, for example, where *Las Parceras* acts as a national network of *acompañante* and the leading feminist advocacy network, *La Mesa Por La Vida*, openly advertises accompaniment as part of its work.

According to activist publications and public conversations, *acompañante* activism is underpinned by a will to be a companion to abortion and abortion seekers (McReynolds-Peréz et al., 2023). As *Red Compañera*, a transnational network of *acompañante* activist groups operating in Latin America and the Caribbean, describe:

> To accompany is to help, is to support, is to give information, is to laugh with them, is to cry with them, is to put together our networks, is to embrace each other, is to hold each other, and this is substantially different when having an abortion experience.

Lux Vacarezza and Burton (2023) conceptualize *acompañante* activism using theories of affect, outlining how networks, many of whom are national-level members of *Red Compañera* such as the Argentinian-based *Socorristas*, Colombia *Parceras* and Mexican *Fondo Maria*, work to create infrastructures of abortion care underpinned by respecting the dignity and voices of abortion seekers. These feminist infrastructures subvert the pre-existing infrastructures available to abortion seekers which are fundamentally characterized by regimes of reproductive governance which discipline and restrict the exercise of reproductive autonomy (Morgan and Roberts, 2012). I will return to this underlying characteristic of *acompañante* activism in later chapters. For now, I want to use *acompañante* activism as exemplifying how abortion trail activism's orientation towards feminist care ethics through maintaining and repairing infrastructures of abortion care so that the abortion experience is characterized by a feminist ethos of reproductive autonomy.

This orientation is reflected in one Colombian *acompañante*'s description of her organization's contribution to abortion care. What is interesting about this activist's account is that it is based on her use of accompaniment networks as an abortion seeker. In her interview, this activist described being provided with information on where to access services, having conversations with *acompañante* on what to expect from the process of taking abortion pills, and being 'partnered' with an activist during the abortion in a private setting. As a user of this infrastructure of abortion care, the respondent felt that her reproductive decisions were respected and not subject to domains of moral, cultural or material policing.

The model of care outlined by this activist resonates with the *Socorristas*' model of accompaniment, published by Zurbriggen, Keefe-Oates and Gerdts in 2018. This 'official' model of accompaniment has four components. To illuminate the similarities between this and a feminist ethic of care practice, I want to detail the first three components in full:

1. A telephone hotline that facilitates initial contact with women. When answering the hotline, *Socorristas* aim to calm anxieties, provide assurances, work through fears, affirm decisions, listen without judgement and strategize situations of violence. During

this initial contact, a group meeting is scheduled where women in need of abortions will meet with several *Socorristas*;
2. In-person group meetings which seek to highlight the collective aspect of the abortion experience and demonstrate that abortions are not solely an individual act but rather something that happens, and can happen, to many women. The *Socorristas* provide women with informational materials created by the *Socorrista* network that describe step-by-step how to use medication to safely induce an abortion;
3. Telephone support during the process of a medication abortion. Telephone support is provided by a *Socorrista* who was present during the group meeting, enabling a personal connection between the woman and the *Socorrista* who is supporting her.

Elsewhere, I have written (with colleagues Cordelia Freeman and Sandra Castaneda Rodriguez) describing *acompañante* activism as a feminist infrastructure of abortion care which is collective, holistic and outside the State (Duffy, Freeman and Rodriguez, 2023). In terms of what the *Socorristas'* model of care indicates about accompaniment, the commitment to collective and holistic care-full feminist infrastructures is obvious. Abortion seekers do not have to explain, justify or apologize for the reproductive choices. However, what is equally clear, is that accompaniment and *acompañante* activism is not necessarily entering into a space of absence. There is – and always was – an infrastructure of abortion in the countries where *acompañante* activism has emerged. But this shadow infrastructure was frequently subject to hyperactive anti-abortion law and policy; emblematic of reproductive structural violence (Nandagiri, Coast and Strong, 2020). As noted in the previous chapter, abortion was inaccessible to many. The formal abortion infrastructures available resulted in coerced and constrained abortion trajectories (Coast et al., 2018), which Freeman, Calkin and others address through the abortion mobilities paradigm.

What is interesting about both the *Socorrista* model of accompaniment, as outlined by Zurbriggen et al., and the account from the *parcera* in Colombia, is that neither account necessarily projects an image of these activists as *constructing* infrastructures of care within an infrastructural void. Indeed, the interviewee in Colombia very clearly outlines how in her first abortion experience she accessed an abortion by way of an infrastructure – an assemblage of objects, things, people and practices. What distinguished this experience from her abortion experience when supported by an *acompañante* infrastructure of care, was that the former abortion was, in her words, 'stigmatizing' and 'violent'. It was also unclear and required self-navigation along often confusing and clandestine pathways, an experience common to that of abortion seekers living in countries like Peru (Duffy, Freeman and Rodriguez, 2023). Similarly, the *Socorristas* have been careful to remind the public that theirs is not the first or original abortion infrastructure. Women access abortion in Argentina without their support; infrastructures of abortion care pre-date the *Socorristas*. The difference between both infrastructures, returning to Corwin and Gidwani (2021) and writing on repair and maintenance by scholars like Strebel (Stebel, Borvet and Sormani, 2018), is that one is limited, fragile, fragmented and precarious and the other is attended to, facilitative and actively sustained. As my colleagues and I commented based on the Peruvian context, *acompañante* activism reflects an infrastructure of care. However, it is important to clarify that the work of the *Socorristas* and *acompañante* activism is not directed at creating an infrastructure of abortion care in the absence of any infrastructure. It is to repair the infrastructure of abortion care as it presently exists so that it is more care-full and equitable. *Socorrisma* and accompaniment offer a *feminist* infrastructure of abortion care which is maintained and repaired through the work of dedicated collectives of activists. These activists engage in tasks and engagements, including providing informational material and assisting planning women's abortion journeys, which smooth over the multiple barriers to abortion that abortion seekers regularly encounter.

The dedication to repairing the available infrastructure of care so that it is both facilitative and care-full is expressed by and visible in the work of abortion trail activists in our places and points in history. The description of a US-based activist working with a national network indicates this dedication:

> There are three things we provide. I think one thing that is overlooked is reassurance. A lot of people are very very overwhelmed, stressed out so the ability we have is to be able to say hey we will provide flights a hotel we will provide contact throughout this process. I think that is a huge part of our service. The other thing is financial support and that can look like a lot of different things but that can look like transportation, meals, hotel – things that you would practically need to get to your care. And then I guess the third ties into the first which is emotional support is something we definitely provide. I think that we all have longer intakes because we want to give people the time to talk to us and we are currently in the process of trying to get a social worker on board so we can have more of that support that we can connect to our clients. (Abortion trail activist, United States, TN102)

This account is instructive when read beside the data and writing on and by Latin American *acompañantes*. While the exact model of care is very different – the US activist helps abortion seekers attend clinics and there are no collective sessions discussing abortion included in their work – the underlying focus of their work resonates with the contribution of *acompañante* activists. Their priority is not necessarily creating an infrastructure but improving and repairing the infrastructure available to abortion seekers. Often this involves what this activist terms as 'reassurance' but, looked at closely, mirrors feminist accompaniment as outlined by both the *Socorristas* and *Red Compañera*. It also involves supporting abortion seekers navigate transport systems as well as, where possible for a group with limited funding, absorbing or minimizing the financial barriers within abortion care infrastructures. In both examples, the work of abortion trail activists is to tend to the infrastructure available to care seekers so the experience of that infrastructure is felt as more supportive and less violent.

Accounts provided by activists in the Netherlands interviewed support an understanding of abortion trail activism as committed to the repair and maintenance of feminist infrastructures of care. As in the United States, there is an infrastructure of abortion care available to both residents and those travelling from abroad in public and private facilities in the Netherlands. Legally, the Netherlands has one of the most liberal abortion care regimes in Europe and a well-developed health service infrastructure. At the same time, activists who participated in the study argued that the infrastructures of abortion care available needed to be maintained consistently and required repair work in places to ensure care remained equitable. They drew particular attention to the infrastructures for those either travelling for abortion care or migrants living in the Netherlands accessing abortion care who did not speak Dutch as a first language. As the activist below comments, abortion trail activists have had to maintain and repair the infrastructures of abortion care to address the disadvantages faced by migrants within the Dutch system:

> And abortion care is basically a whole separate law that is still actually in the law illegal but there is exceptions which makes it illegal. So yeah, I think it is like in a lot of places like this abortion legislation is still a very obscure law. Where there just like a lot of things that are still kind of illegal but they are because we just don't talk about. For example, like in the Dutch legislation, this is the law but no one really knows about it. So we try to collaborate with other organisations to talk to also the Union of Abortion Care Workers that this is the situation and you know please acknowledge and inform your clinics and it had very little resonance actually. Also because basically what we heard from them is basically that we don't get these clients. Which is just not true because, yeah, they don't get these clients because they turn them away. They turn them away at reception and then yeah, they don't get these clients. (Abortion trail activist, the Netherlands, TN103)

The comments of US- and Netherlands'-based abortion trail activists are interesting as they point to a will to repair and maintain feminist infrastructures of abortion. This can mean developing new connections with different parts of the overarching abortion care infrastructure or infrastructural adaptations. Theorists working on caring infrastructures, repair and maintenance through a feminist ethic of care lens note how changing infrastructural components in response to challenges reported by those in positions where the infrastructure results in unequal treatment is a quintessential reflection of feminist ethic of care practice. This commitment to repairing and maintaining infrastructures to avoid inequities is visible in the work of US- and Netherlands-based abortion trail activists. It manifests in actions like reaching out to clinic staff or establishing funding programmes for additional transportation costs accrued by those, living in countries like the United States, who increasingly cannot access services locally.

Comparing these accounts with those from research participants in other jurisdictions, in Africa for example, we see a similar commitment to repairing/maintaining infrastructures so that they are consistent with a feminist care ethic present in the work of abortion trail activists. Let us take, for example, the comments of the activist below on their personal experience of witnessing the broken infrastructures of abortion care during their own training as a midwife:

> Okay, so I started training as a nurse/midwife in the mid-1980s when we still had the previous abortion law in [country] which was very restrictive, and I came across a number of septic abortions and they fundamentally challenged me, and at the same time I was witness to some of my peers accessing private services and going to [country]. So, I had that experience and in particular saw very poor racialised treatment of women in being kind of scolded and neglected, at the same time there was such a burden of septic abortions that the wards were segregated, white and black wards, and at one stage they actually had to use some of the white wards for black women. I remember once being allocated to a white ward that there were four black women in that ward with septic abortions and that in a sense was a compounded issue because they were deviant in having septic abortions and they were deviant in desegregating the hospitals. (Activist, Africa, WA110)

Again, the activist points to the existence of an infrastructure of abortion care which is moralistic, restrictive and disrespectful of abortion seekers' reproductive decision-making. It was also, in this context, racialized. Fundamentally, they describe an infrastructure of care in need of significant repair. At the same time, the point remains that an infrastructure existed, it was just, as elucidated by this personal account, almost wholly problematic. The role of abortion trail activism within this context was to repair the infrastructure of abortion care, often through mundane and granular activities as this activist continues:

> I then probably made an unconscious political commitment to redress these things that I saw and it has been something that I've felt as I kind of cared for those women. So, washing them, kind of taking their temperature, when nobody else would go in and they'll be neglected, making sure that their antibiotics were on time. (Activist, Africa, WA110)

While the work of this African activist was markedly different from the work of activists in the Netherlands or the United States, all three are underpinned by a similar commitment – to ensuring the infrastructure of abortion care operates according to feminist principles.

Conclusions

> caring is full of both problems and possibilities. Caring for others can be a source of pleasure and fulfillment, but it can also be undervalued and denied, a source of degradation and exploitation. Care not only exists within intimate relationships but is also located within global-scale hierarchies of gender, class and race/ethnicity. Care can be problematic for those who need it, who give it and who arrange care for others, but it can also be the most precious thing in the world to them. (Cox, 2010: 113)

The work of abortion trail activists detailed in this chapter speaks to a further characterizing commitment of their work to ensuring abortion's accessibility – a commitment to a non-normative feminist ontological model of abortion care. This manifests in two ways. First, it results in efforts to normalize abortion and reinforce its ontological position as both an essential form of care and part of the social and cultural fabric of the societies within which the abortion trail activists operate. Second, it is enacted through work which aims to address problematic and inequitable infrastructures of abortion care many abortion seekers have to resort to. These infrastructures frequently need to be navigated by abortion seekers without support, do not respect reproductive autonomy, are riven with restrictions and result in feelings of stigma as well as excessive financial burdens. Pursuing a feminist ethic of care, abortion trail activists work to repair, and where necessary maintain, abortion care infrastructures in adherence with feminist principles of care.

Including repair and maintenance work within our definition of abortion trail activism broadens the discussion of what abortion trail activism contributes to the project of abortion access beyond the creation of mechanisms for accessing abortion. Most importantly, it demonstrates that the interventions of activists and support they provide are political acts rather than functional responses.

3

Prefiguring Abortion Infrastructures

Introduction

The previous chapters have outlined the commitments that orientate the work of abortion trail activists. While the data can only ever provide an indication, looking across the accounts of activists in different jurisdictions, regions and at different points in time, it is possible to identify shared concerns of abortion trail activism. Based on research informing this book, I have identified accessibility, a will to establish a non-normative ontological understanding of abortion care and an effort to repair and maintain infrastructures of abortion care so they reflect feminist principles as common goals. By discussing the goals of abortion trail activist collectives, these chapters expand on existing literature considering abortion trails through paradigms of travel and mobilities. They also emphasized the ontological nature of abortion care that abortion trails amplify while highlighting, through drawing attention to the phenomenological attitude demonstrated by activists as well as their orientation of pre-existing care subjectivities and routeways (e.g. aunties) towards disrupting impediments to abortion, that their activism is clearly emblematic of a political project rather than a functional or civil response.

Having identified these as shared characteristics of abortion trail activism, I now want to locate abortion trail activism within the broader spectrum of political activism. Following Vivaldi and Stutzin (2021) and Pierson (2023), the chapter presents abortion trail activism as a form of prefigurative politics which, as already outlined, is committed to an ethics of feminist care and accessibility. I argue, using primary and secondary data, that this theoretical model captures the political ideology driving abortion trail activism despite the varied structure, size and engagements of movements in different places, spaces and times. Through prefiguration, I also try to bridge abortion trail activism with side-along political praxes which are prefigurative without defining abortion trail activism as a manifestation of these other political forms entirely. Specifically, I draw attention to health social movement activism and reproductive justice.

My objective here, developing Lin et al. (2016)'s arguments about engendering prefigurative politics (within which the authors connect reproductive justice and prefigurative politics), is to bridge prefigurative politics with the spirit of these movements in a way that allows us to recognize the prefigurative character of abortion trail activism more deeply, that values the practices as political of abortion trail activists in and of themselves, and that appreciates the tensions and contestations within abortion trail activism. In other words, I want to be able to talk about the politics of abortion trail activism without constructing abortion trail activism as having a master epistemology, casting abortion trail activism as having no distinguishable political ideology, or overlooking its complexity. This second component of the chapter's discussion will form the basis of the next part of this book where I consider how a direct engagement with abortion trail activism enriches our understanding of the objectives of and contestations within the global pro-choice project.

Understanding prefigurative politics

The term prefigurative politics was first coined by Boggs (1977) as an alternative exercise of leftist politics built on a criticism of Marxist politics as separating the goal of constructing an alternative social order from the present conduct of leftist social transformation projects. Broadly writ, prefigurative politics argues that the construction of alternative futures through social movement organizing needs to manifest within or in parallel with present conduct and action within and by social movements (Yates, 2015). Boggs' political imagining originally focused predominantly on the projects for State or macro-level transformation and attempted to construct a model of political praxis that avoided the observable dissonance, also highlighted by Marxist feminists such as Federici, between the micro-level quotidian actions within social movements and their stated political objectives. The core complaint inspiring prefigurative politics was the necessity of openly recognizing and actively challenging 'how people in movements for social justice often relate to each other in oppressive ways' (Cornish et al., 2016: 115). The path to anti-hierarchical social transformation, for commentators like Boggs, could not be achieved by mobilizations which, in their conduct, did not subvert the established hierarchical social order.

Theoretically, this is consistent with anarchist, particularly anarchofeminist and avante-garde political theory which advocates a total and consistent disruption of social order across scales of social and political engagement as essential to broader social transformation. It also resonated with challenges to leftist political organizing and dominant orthodoxies of oppression raised by feminist thinkers like Federici and Black feminist scholars like Angela K. Davis. Arguably, Boggs was not necessarily the 'founder' of prefigurative politics but was instead articulating, through this concept, a critique against the 'Old Left' (i.e. Marxist movements) for ignoring lived oppressions, including oppressions within leftism, in pursuit of a 'larger' struggle. This can explain why, as Cornish et al. (2016) write,

> The term was embraced by feminism, anarchism and the New Left to bring into focus modes of practice that make it possible to envision a transformed society based on actual human capacities rather than abstract principles (Boggs, 1977). These movements were guided by the idea that radical social change requires creating and experimenting with the kinds of egalitarian practices, democratic spaces, and

alternative modes of relating that anticipate a future society that cannot yet be fully realized . (Cornish et al., 2016: 115)

Prefigurative politics has been since read as social transformation through modes of political action which do not delineate between future and present. Critical legal theorists such as Grabham (2016) offer a useful phrasing of this argument through their writing on how practices 'brew' social order and offer meaningful, lived improvement. This includes mutual aid, co-operative movements and the creation of spaces of economic and environmental/ecological alterity all of which challenge neoliberal political order through everyday, often experimental, ways of relating to each other. These practices, according to the logics of prefigurative politics, ultimately facilitate meaningful social transformation as they gain recognition of sustainable, continuous forms of social improvement. As Spade (2020), writing on mutual aid, argues, prefigurative political action is essential to ensuring that the material, lived experience of society is actually disrupted by social movements which present themselves as intent on social justice reform. Spade critiques the 'Old Left' position of social justice movements inevitably resulting in social transformation, as he notes in the following quote:

> Many reforms provide no material relief and change only what the system says about itself, such as when institutions pass antidiscrimination policies but nothing about the behavior of participants or the outcomes of their operations change. (Spade, 2020: 132)

Emphasizing both the material present and the potential for leftist/social justice–orientated movements to overlook, and thus permit the persistence of, lived oppression is an important, and certainly repeated, theme within Black, anti-colonial/decolonial and anti-racist writing. In *Sister Outsider*, Audre Lorde writes openly about her experience of being silenced within White feminist campaigns for drawing attention to the forms of injustice, including epistemic violence which erased Black histories, the master project of feminist politics was ignoring. Similarly, in *Women, Race and Class*, Angela Y. Davis underlined how racialized material inequality was neglected, and often reinforced by, feminist social justice movements. More recently, the decolonial scholars Yang and Tuck (2021) have drawn attention to the failure of anti-racist and supposed decolonizing movements to meaningfully address colonial, racialized oppression by treating the decolonizing project as a 'metaphor'.

At the same time, social justice writing has pushed back against calls for prefigurative engagements through questioning whether presentist work which disrupts uneven and unjust social order actually can or does result in fundamental, long-lasting change. The question here is, at base, whether quotidian action which offers a space of alterity or addresses material inequalities is facilitating the desired social transformation that Boggs argued needed to run in parallel with prefigurative action. In other words, if we transform the present to transform the future, do we actually transform the future? There is ample evidence, based on the experiments of the 1970s and 1980s, that prefigurative politics does not result in system change. We still, after all, live in a world characterized by the forms of oppression that anarchist and feminist movements which embraced prefiguration claimed the 'Old Left' was ignoring.

To an extent, this pushback is contrarian and it is possible to fall into a 'tyranny of the empirical' (Cornish et al., 2016: 115) where prefigurative political projects are dismissed because we have not observably, to date, transformed society. That said, there are important issues raised in critiques of prefiguration. Predominant among these is the risk of co-optation by elites of actions that aim to challenge lived experiences of material, embodied and political inequality as part of a more expansive project of shoring up neoliberal political systems through deflecting attention away from structural problems. There is certainly a risk, by presenting material need and relational exclusion as essential to social transformation, to enable political elites to present themselves as committed to social transformation by addressing these problems. This strategy is emblematized by phenomena such as 'pink washing', 'greenwashing', 'sport washing' and 'astroturfing' where multinational, neoliberal corporate bodies will engage with lived oppressed in small, everyday but meaningful ways (for the individuals or communities) and then use these engagements in marketing strategies which cast them as harmless or even benevolent.

The root of this co-optation is the overuse of prefiguration as a descriptor for all political interventions focused on present concerns. As Gordon (2018) notes, the term can be used too extensively, leading to organizations who are focused on presentist issues becoming labelled prefigurative. There is an important difference between these two, often co-existent, political practices. Presentism means to focus on addressing injustice in the here and now; prefiguration means undertaking modes of political action and mobilization which bring forth – in the here and now – an imagined future where injustice is lessened or absent into being. Presentism means dealing with the immediate needs *of* the present moment; prefiguration means *future-making* in and through actions *in* the present moment.

Critiques of prefigurative politics from social movement studies and in Gordon's writing, rightly, highlight the risk of disconnecting transformation in and of the present from the ongoing or future project of social transformation. The issue here is that, by emphasizing the need to make progress on including and challenging the oppressions experienced by marginalized voices, and focusing attentions on this work, social movements may fall behind on the 'macro'-level or structural challenges. Furthermore, the orientation to challenging oppression at the margins may result in the persistence of 'rescue work' (Haaken, 2010) discourses which construct marginalized and oppressed subjects as inherently outside, vulnerable and oppressed. These discourses, as theorists such as Spivak and Chandra Mohanty have consistently underlined, impede marginalized subjects from gaining recognition of, or indeed the space to engage in, work which challenges the oppression they experience without being 'rescued'.

Advocates of prefigurate politics such as Sara Motta (2017) contend that the way through these problematics is through centring both the logics underpinning prefiguration as a project and practices that are reflective of prefigurative politics. Global South theory offers useful analytic tools for this centring as it emphasizes critical reflection and critical pedagogy by movements on *movements* as well as by movements on *social relations*. Prefigurative politics is a combination of reflection and action – a praxis – where movements weave together theory and practice about how systems of power operate and persist and how both the operation and persistence of power can be meaningfully disrupted. Critically, prefigurative politics must engage with the lived present and its historic foundations without tying itself to a specific configuration of what a most just social order looks like imagined in the present. To connect oneself to an imagined future, as Ahmed (2020) and Berlant (2007) outline, is to suspend a future on the present. Doing so produces sets of subject relations which may neither be just nor anti-oppressive as our imaginings of the future are influenced by the social order as we understand it at this point in time. These imaginings can, as Swatuk and Vale (2016) note, valorize a pre-capitalist 'golden age' (which was equally oppressive but in different ways) or a 'better' way of doing statist governance (which is largely modelled on the capitalist state).

Central to prefigurative politics is a distancing from a politics of 'counterstance' without reducing itself to mutual aid. Prefigurative politics sees the former as more problematic than the latter. As Anzaldúa (1987) writes in relation to a social justice politics built solely on counterstance critiques of dominant social orders (like Marxism but also feminist arguments than do not address lived injustice in the present):

> It is not enough to stand on the opposite river bank, shouting questionings, challenging patriarchal, white conventions. A counterstance locks one into a duel of oppressor and oppressed; locked in as mortal combat, like the cop and the criminal, both are reduced to a common denominator of violence, The counterstance refutes the dominant culture's views and beliefs, and, for this, it is proudly defiant. All reaction is limited by, and dependent on, what it is reacting against. (Anzaldúa, 1987: 78)

Anzaldúa's argument, expressed through her theory of Chicana feminism, is that we need to look for and engage with transformative politics using the resources available to us rather than delaying transformation until the outright dismantling of the state has been achieved. At the same time, according to Anzaldúa and others, it is possible to weave a liberation (Motta, 2018) and disruption of state power through quotidian transformative practices.

Equally, prefigurative politics also resists casting practices of mutual aid, disconnected from a broader political project, to transformation. It is worth noting here that 'practices of mutual aid' are different to mutual aid politics which, as Spade (2020) emphasizes, must be connected with a substance critique and ongoing effort to disrupt political systems which have emerged within and are sustained by capitalist, colonialist and neoliberal discourses. The critical point here, as the aforementioned arguments regarding 'presentism' (Gordon) allude to, is that prefigurative politics rejects the presentation of action outside or distinct from statist practices as inherently progressive. Prefigurative political transformation is a praxis; it is only meaningfully progressive if the work is embedded within and engages with the discursively produced systems of power which restrict, control and actively police bodies and selves.

Prefigurative politics' arguments are derived from its conceptual underpinnings – particularly critical pedagogy, critical theory and Black/socialist feminist theory. Each of these foreground three things. First, the importance of building political transformation from disrupting the lived experience of uneven power relations which have been produced by colonial, capitalist and neoliberal discourses within the context of those discourses. Second, the need to remain open to the potential for discourse to become radically altered in unpredictable ways if we practice a critique of the dominant social order in our everyday relationships and ways of thinking about ourselves. Third, the centrality of critical education and both learning and unlearning established knowledges, including those knowledges established by social justice movements.

In their work on prefiguration, gender and reproductive justice, Lin et al. (2016) synthesize prefigurative politics' core principles to three pursuits – challenging relationality, addressing intersectional oppressions and facilitating self-determination. These authors characterize prefigurative politics as a praxis that pursues social transformation through collective, anti-oppressive ways of relating to each other; strategies that recognize and address co-existing and intersecting injustices; and infrastructures that remove the requirement to seek permission or legitimacy from another actor (i.e. the State). Importantly, they decouple prefigurative politics from the achievement of a more just society. Their argument here is influenced by the original position of prefigurative writing – that oppression can exist and persist within the confines of socially transformative work. As Lin et al. write, prefigurative politics 'is not something we create to call in a future without (or nostalgically *before*) oppression and violence but rather *in spite of* (Lin et al., 2016: 305; italics in original).

Having provided a brief outline of prefigurative politics, I now want to connect this lens with the work of abortion trail activists. In doing so, as I set out in the introduction to this chapter, I want to offer a way of understanding and recognizing abortion trail activism as political. By reading abortion trail activism as prefigurative politics, I argue that it is possible to avoid disconnecting abortion trail activist mobilizations from each other because they have different structures or engage in different practices. Equally, working with prefigurative politics, it is possible to locate abortion trail activism within the broader landscape of political action which runs alongside it – specifically reproductive justice and health social movement activism. Having established a vehicle for understanding what orientates abortion trail activism, I will conclude by identifying the threads that the second part of this book will revisit.

Reading abortion trail activism as prefigurative

It is really interesting because there is a philosophical question here that I have been spending a lot of time thinking about and talking about a lot with colleagues of mine outside of ORGANISATION who also do practical support. We need to define practical support but how do you define something that is just human existence? (Abortion trail activist, United States, TN103)

What we do is accompany with love.... Working not only from theory but from practice.... We promote access to information and to care as a political principle... against medical hegemony. (Sutton, 2021)

Prefiguration has been increasingly used in literature considering the distinct qualities of the Latin American feminist movements, specifically those focused on abortion and gender-based violence, that have emerged since the early 2000s. A key marker of women's struggles in Latin America at the current moment, as Gustá writes, is that they are prefigurative 'which means challenging patriarchy in everyday life' (Gustá, 2021). As Gustá describes:

[These movements] develop performative and cultural actions aimed at a symbolic transformation of the gendered order [. . .] Prefigurative actions can also take the form of activists providing support for battered women and for women seeking abortion.

Vivaldi and Stutzin (2021) also point to the prefigurative spirit of Latin American feminist activism on abortion. The prefigurative nature of this activism is reflected in their concern for creating a new way of seeing abortion in the present moment through direct action and the creation of infrastructures of abortion care (Duffy, Freeman and Castañeda, 2023).

Importantly, these prefigurative infrastructures of abortion care – *acompañante* activism – are shaped by and emblematize an active critique of both the infrastructures and constructions of abortion formed by and within discourses of reproductive health in the Latin American space. These are not solely alternative modes of accessing abortion; they are an enacted resistance to the construction of abortion as an individual, moral failure which should be difficult and traumatic so that it does not become accepted. This resistance is at the same time a reworking of the affective experience of abortion (Vacarezza and Burton, 2023) and an active, persistent remembering of the role of State infrastructures and logics, specifically those informed by transnational politics of reproductive health (which emphasized family planning) and representational politics of gendered respectability (see also Skeggs, 1997), in sustaining an imagining of abortion as undesirable and requiring eradication. These State infrastructures included medical architectures which approached abortion through a biomedical curative logic rather than a feminist ethic of care that, as noted in the preceding chapter, saw abortion as ontological.

The characterization of activists providing support – through *acompañante* activism – as prefigurative are clearly significant in terms of reading abortion trail activism as exemplary of prefigurative politics. Its accuracy is further reinforced by comments from *acompañantes* and Latin American abortion activists regarding both their aspiration and their daily work to transform how those who abort and who seek abortion are treated in the Latin American space (as typified in the quote from Valeria Vergas, a member of *Red Compañera*, at the beginning of this section). While both the aptness of prefiguration to describing abortion trail activisms in Latin America and the established connection between these feminisms and prefigurative politics in literature reassuringly support my reading of abortion trail activism as prefigurative, they do present a number of analytic challenges.

First, there is the temptation to impose the forms of abortion activism read as prefigurative in literature on Latin America to all abortion trail activism. This potential results in conflating the practices of activists in one space, place and time with the underpinning objectives and aspirations of those activists. The aspiration of abortion activists in Latin America is not best read as an aspiration to create artistic representations, but an aspiration to fundamentally disrupt the position of abortion within the broader gendered, anti-abortion discourse through collective representations of abortion as desired, desirable, joyous and loving. It pursues an infrastructure of abortion disconnected from the medical profession as there is an established history of the use of health services to achieve political projects underpinned by reproductive governance.

The second challenge that the established reading of Latin American abortion feminisms as prefigurative politics brings is that, because of the particularities of how prefigurative politics manifests in this context, it disconnects Latin America from other movements. These movements, as I will describe in this section, offer examples of prefigurative action which create 'desired alternatives or utopian visions for a fairer, freer, and more sustainably-balanced world through the actions, practices and social relationships they build in the here and now' (Habersang, 2022: 2). The key challenge is to recognize work that involves sustainable social and political transformation and which enables greater autonomy and self-determination for those who occupy a position of 'non-being' (Motta, 2018) through relational practices and collective actions in the present as prefigurative if it does not take the forms commonly found in Latin America.

Consistent with this delineation, I want to draw on very different accounts of actions by abortion trail activists that can, through Lin et al.'s (2016) definition be read as prefigurative politics as opposed to a counterstance. The first is from an African activist:

> [Activists in organisation] work with the community health workers but also the peer educators within the communities so that they're able to identify some of these young girls who have experienced this. Now, I mean, I think that's a lengthy process in terms of being able to know who requires the service but in most cases, most of these community health workers might know the information around you know, how many teens are pregnant in the community.
>
> So through that, community health workers identify these different young girls and they work with the families to identify are the families willing to go ahead and consent or provide guidance or authorisation that these children can actually, actually they are children yes, and what they can really provide to get that service. So, you will find that you know, those who are already identified are already from poor backgrounds, those who probably didn't complete school, whose

parents don't have any income, and so what they do is they really accompany them from wherever they are to the health centre and they're able to connect them with the health centres, as you know find all the papers. (Activist, Africa E202)

Set against the ways of acting that typify current abortion trail activism within the Latin American space, there is little to suggest a shared political praxis. The account above does not describe collective creative interventions which radically reimagine the embodied or affective experience of abortion. However, while the practices outlined by the African activist do not resonate with those documented in research on Latin America, there are aspects that speak to prefigurative labours.

For example, the respondent talks about collaborating with community health workers, peer educators and families to reduce the barriers to abortion women and girls encounter. There are visible echoes here with the prefigurative ideal outlined by Lin et al. of building new worlds through collective, relational activities. In this instance, the actors involved in the relationship are different to those in the Latin American space – instead of large groups of feminist activists, the African activist above identifies a network of relations involving community health workers, local educators and families. Yet the alternative abortion landscape they are working to create is the same as activists in Latin America; African activists direct their efforts to reducing the alienation felt by abortion seekers, the exclusion of their bodies from spaces of health and care and the treatment of their health desires as less acceptable.

Moreover, again resonating with Latin American prefigurative interventions, activists in the African space are keenly aware of, and conscious to both highlight and challenge, the uneven economics of abortion. Through their work, which addresses the immediate financial burden of abortion and provides support to remedy the forms of cultural and epistemic capital (e.g. understanding of legal rights, ability to complete clinic paperwork), they also emphasize and disrupt the socio-economic hierarchies that inflect abortion care in their communities.

These hierarchies were explicitly challenged by one activist working in Africa:

> I think what will happen now is that you have people who have the money, and you have people who don't have the money. If you have, it's the same old story that all the countries know, if you have the money you can fly to whichever country around that has the abortion and has doctors, because some people have the law, but you still don't have any doctors to do it, but some places they have doctors who will do it and do it well. (Activist, Africa E102)

As another respondent, working in a different part of Africa, highlighted, one of their core areas of work was rebalancing the economics of abortion so that less privileged women were also able to access care. This activist, along with activists in other African countries, highlighted the fact that economic and cultural capital played a significant role in dictating abortion trajectories. Consistent with prefigurative political actions, activists in this space integrated amplifying and educating others about these inequalities within their work as outlined in the quote below:

> We talk about it as something that we need to advocate for and we reached a point of categorising it as a class issue. It may not affect someone who is able to gather their money and they go out there to a good private clinic or hospital and they get it, but to someone, that's the other person who is able to access the service will not feel the pain, you know will not understand the intersections of the other women who are in the rural areas, the other women who are from [name of region], from poor backgrounds, they will not understand it. (Activist, Africa, E206)

Again, here we see reflections of prefigurative politics. In Africa, while abortion trail activists do not engage in creative actions, they are practising the same political praxis where critical education is used as a mechanism for transforming how abortion access is thought of (in this instance as a class issue).

The work of activists supporting women travelling from Ireland seeking for abortion, and those seeking abortion on the island of Ireland since the early 2000s, also speak to aspects of prefigurative political action. Similar to the Latin American and African contexts, the history of abortion access for women living in Ireland has been characterized by a combination of State-implemented barriers to care, social isolation and stigma. Anti-abortion sentiment, according to one activist who described their experience of acting as a 'clinic defender' or escort – a form of activist practice which involved standing outside sexual and reproductive health clinics as a barrier between those seeking services and anti-abortion protestors – often manifested in abusive ways, including verbal insults and spitting:

> The first couple of times we did it, it was difficult and it's hard to explain to people how aggressive and unsettling those interactions were. You were on a public highway or public street and there would be somebody this close to your face, shouting at the top of their voice. Erm, even though it wasn't necessarily about us it became, the longer we were there, the longer it became about us, but at the start it was just about what we represented. It was still an incredibly erm difficult to deal with interaction publicly and I think that's why they did it because you're in front of the public it is public shaming [. . .] And seeing how shaken and how frightened people were coming in and how frightened they were. (Activist, Northern Ireland)

To address the social acts of exclusion, including the violent protests described in this quote, abortion trail activists supporting women living in and travelling from Ireland for abortion worked to construct an affective experience of abortion as characterized by emotional support and respect. This is illustrated in the quote below from an interview with two activists involved in the Liverpool Abortion Support Service:

> I think there was an awareness of how isolated they were [. . .] emotionally and physically in a strange place and it really was to fill that gap to offer them somewhere to stay, someone who would be on their side and non-judgemental and that was a huge thing.

Someone who would listen they had to keep quiet about it so often. (Activists, LASS6)

The quotes above do not speak solely to acts of kindness or attempts to protect abortion seekers from public shaming. They were part of a broader orientation towards disrupting and reconstructing the experience of abortion as one which was characterized by protection and emotional support. According to writing on what constitutes prefiguration (Lin et al., 2016), the will to transform experiences that are reflective of injustice – in this case the public condemnation and social isolation of people making particular reproductive choices – must translate into interventions that actively, albeit incrementally, reconstruct the affective experience of abortion. The quote from an activist involved in ESCORT, an abortion trail activist organization that developed after LASS ceased operations. ESCORT activists also aimed to support people travelling from the island of Ireland to Liverpool for abortions but, as the description of their work suggests, reflects a prefigurative intervention to transform the experience of abortion mobilities (Freeman, 2020) for this marginalized group:

> I would contact the rota of volunteers. I would try to do it fairly as it was people giving up whole weekends of their time. I would contact one of them or for myself to get the flight details and go to the airport and meet the women from the plane. Given them details of what I looked like etc. and this is quite a strong memory because the airport is quite a grim area and women would be coming back late at night because they were travelling at quite unsociable times. Partly because of appointment times but also to save money by getting a ridiculously early or late flights. Then bring them back to our houses and then settle them in . . . food etc. but there was a fasting requirement at the time. Then the next morning we would bring them [clinic's administration and registration office] and either that day usually that day later to the [main clinic] (ESCORT 1).

These examples, while limited in scope, are indicative of the appropriateness of prefigurative politics as a mechanism from foregrounding the shared underlying political ideology of abortion trail activist groups in different jurisdictions. I will return to this point in the next section of this chapter.

At this juncture, it is important to recognize the differences between movements, and indeed the contradictions that emerge when abortion trail activism in different places and spaces are framed as politically resonate. There are irrefutable distinctions between, for example, abortion trail activism in Latin America and the Caribbean and in the African space. In relation to abortion trail activism in these jurisdictions, a key difference is the extent of collaboration with health care professionals by abortion trail activists in Africa as opposed to their Latin American counterparts who, as Sutton (2021) argues, aim to challenge the presence of the medical establishment in the abortion experience. In drawing attention to this difference, I want to further appraise whether prefigurative politics can be applied to abortion trail activism which engages in practices diverging from those in the Latin American space.

In the African context, groups whose work I have depicted as speaking to prefigurative and transformative aims as they work to construct ways of relating to and supporting abortion seekers which challenge dominant discourses of abortion often collaborate with health care professionals. These collaborations include values clarification and legal education sessions with health workers to establish what the World Health Organization (2022) describes as an enabling environment for abortion to exist. They also include training health workers on abortion procedures and establishing networks of community health workers who can provide abortion services in marginalized communities (including townships and rural areas).

Viewed through the lens of Latin American abortion activism, there is a tension between these collaborations and the political praxis of prefigurative feminist accompaniment. A core principle of prefigurative abortion politics as interpreted by groups like *Red Compañera*, is the need to resist the biomedicalization of abortion as something that requires involvement of medical professionals. The rationale behind this resistance is derived from an opposition to medical hegemony which has contributed to reproductive governance (Duffy, Freeman and Castañeda, 2023) combined with a commitment to the demedicalization of abortion (Halfmann, 2012) and interpretation of demedicalization as the resting of control over abortion care from health institutions. If we consider resistance to medical hegemony as characteristic of prefigurative political action, as emblematized by Latin American *acompañante* activism, then arguably by actively reaching out to health care professionals African abortion activism self-excludes from the umbrella of prefiguration by default.

However, returning to my earlier point, derived from Anzadúla's (1987) writing, it is essential to avoid reducing projects attempting to transform the present to counterstances. The prefigurative spirit of *acompañante* activism is not embodied in an opposition to health workers' involvement in abortion. Its transformative orientation is representative of an effort to make explicit, through openly challenging, the power relations, inequalities and governing logics that are entangled with abortion health services. Just as we cannot consider all mobilizations which present a different way of delivering the services historically provided by the State as manifestations of prefiguration; we should not present the inclusion of service providers who work within State institutions in mobilizations which are experimenting with different ways of addressing need in the present as necessarily antithetical to prefiguration.

Even in their inclusion of health professionals, the accounts of abortion trail activists in the African space speak to a will to create an alternative future through actions in the present. Their collaborations with health workers indicate that they also recognize that part of that alternative future, and by consequence the presentist efforts to transform, may involve health care workers. At face value, this seems to run counter to the position of Latin American abortion trail activists. However, it is not insignificant that the activists in the African space, through who they engage in these health care professional dialogues, present an understanding of who counts as a health worker that extends beyond the boundaries of biomedical hegemony. While activists interviewed in the research identified medics in hospitals, nurses and pharmacists as health workers who they reached out to as part of their project to expand abortion access, many organizations described community health workers as the main actors within the infrastructures of abortion care their organization aimed to establish. The people who fell under this label included members of the community, community healers as well as midwifes and nurses.

The central point I want to highlight here is that, although there is more reaching out to health professionals in Africa than in Latin America, from the accounts of activists in the African space we can see a similar commitment to constructing an infrastructure of abortion care which supports women seeking abortions in ways that are sensitive to their emotional and physical needs. This commitment is visible in the description by an activist in Africa of how their work to develop an infrastructure of abortion care has developed:

> through our work with pharmacists on referring women to them, we started working with the community health volunteers because they are very closely attached to the women and girls in their villages and their communities, so women and girls trust them more, and they are able to tell them 'I need to access safe abortion', and these community health volunteers, we have introduced them to these pharmacists, so on the time when they get a women in the community who wants to access their pills, they escort them to that pharmacist, because sometimes when you send a woman, she'll fear going alone, because maybe she wants somebody to speak on her behalf, and also, we, when we identified the community health risk, the community health volunteers and train them, they're also able to support the women as their providers following up, so the risk of unsafe, we tried to handle that, the risk of the fear of security for these women, we also try to handle because now she's supported, and the risk of also who is attending to her, we were also able to manage to handle that. (Activist, Africa, WA105)

If we recognize both the inclusion and training of community health volunteers, who may not be trained as medics or part of the official medical establishing, as reflective of an orientation towards generating infrastructures of abortion care that challenge the position of medics as directors of reproductive health experiences, then the prefigurative political character of African abortion activism becomes more visible. Like activisms in the Latin American space, there is an argument for characterizing the work to construct, repair and maintain abortion trails (outlined in the previous chapter) as representative of a particular political project underpinned by prefiguration.

Conclusions

This chapter has presented abortion trail activism as a reflective of prefigurative politics. In doing so, it has offered a conceptual model for connecting the commitments discussed in the preceding chapter with a wider political project. It has also shown, through reading abortion trail activism in different jurisdictions through the lens of prefiguration, the possibility of discussing seemingly incomparable forms of activist work as underpinned by a mutually resonant political ideology. What does thinking about abortion trail activism as a prefigurative politics contribute to our understanding of these activisms? The section above has indicated how a prefigurative lens allows us to consider mobilizations that are very different in terms of their strategies and engagements as politically similar. Here I want to consider how associating abortion trail activism with this political framing progresses the conversation about this form of activism forwards. Again, my objective here is to move our conceptualization and understanding of abortion trail activism from empirical descriptions of individual movements towards an appreciation of abortion trail activism as a political intervention underpinned by specific concerns and ideological projects.

This undertaking emerged from conversations with activists in organizations engaged in abortion trail work. While they could eloquently outline the focus of their work, eliciting an appropriate banner for their organization was more challenging. Many connected themselves with coalitions supporting abortion access through facilitating abortion travel, distributing abortion pills, offering information or financing abortion seekers. These self-definitions – as parceras, practical support groups, sexual and reproductive health networks, or abortion support networks – partly reflect the context organizations operated in. They also broadly summarize the work of abortion trail activist groups. Yet, as this and the preceding chapters highlight, to ensure that a description of work does not dominate the discussion of abortion trail activism, it is important to consider the underlying commitments and political projects that this work connects to. The question here, which this first part of the book has sought to address, is what do we find if we talk about abortion trail work as an activism which can be, and has been, practised in differing ways?

Following this intellectual exercise has drawn attention to shared commitments and politics that we can connect with abortion trail activism – a commitment to accessibility and a feminist ethic of care as well as a prefigurative political praxis. My question now is what the last element – prefiguration – brings to the project of theorizing abortion trail activism beyond individual actions taken at particular moments in time, in specific locations. To conclude this chapter and assist the transition to the second part of this book, I want to home in on three benefits of considering abortion trail activism as prefigurative politics.

First, prefiguration, as noted already in this chapter, removes the need to delineate organizations based on the scope or scale of their work. If we appreciate groups as similarly intent on constructing a presentist imaginary of a desired futurity, then the substance of their activities becomes less of a differentiating marker. This is important in the context of abortion trail activism where there is a temptation to categorize organizations who are orientated towards resonant prefigurative political goals as markedly dissimilar. Foregrounding prefiguration as a driving force draws attention to the shared political ideologies of mobilizations which, on first sight, appear incomparable. There are clear benefits to this analytically as it removes the problem of separating out organizations based on the specificities of their work or membership, a process which ignores or does not appreciate the reality that abortion trail activism may include a wide range of actors. Through prefiguration, we can move away from an understanding of abortion trails as always existing outside or in complete isolation from health services – an understanding that overlooks the contribution of and collaboration with community health workers, pharmacists and health care providers. Prefiguration here allows us to discuss abortion trail activism as a capacious political intervention as opposed to an alternative label for discrete types of activist group (e.g. practical support networks, abortion pills activists, hosting collectives and so on).

The second benefit of adding prefiguration to discussions regarding the qualities of abortion trail activism is that it enables theoretical conversations to meaningfully consider the differences and similarities between abortion trail activism and other forms of reproductive, care and health activism. Again, this benefit is rooted in the interpretation of abortion trail activism as praxis – theory and action – as opposed to solely function. The main contribution of prefiguration is that we are better able to identify what distinguishes abortion trail activism from, or indeed what connects it to, other gendered and embodied health social movements, such as the breast cancer movement, the birth rights movement or patient advocacy movements (Brown, 2004). If abortion trail activism is prefigurative, then it is political and intent on establishing a transformative imagining of abortion in the present rather than campaigning or engendering improvements in abortion in the future. If we accept that premise, then we are better able to separate the politics that abortion trail activism pursues from other political mobilizations for health. Using prefiguration, it is possible to explore, in a similar vein to Roberts et al.'s (2016) work on health social movements and cause regimes, the contestations that have emerged as the 'causes' of abortion trail activism (i.e. improving abortion care, addressing barriers to access) have shifted over time and as the movements themselves have evolved.

We are equally able to reflect on the position of abortion trail activism within the political movement for reproductive justice. As numerous activists, scholars and scholar-activists have noted, reproductive justice emerged out of a critique of the centring of abortion rights by liberal pro-choice advocacy. Coalitions like SisterSong have persistently highlighted the need to adopt a broader view of how reproductive rights and autonomy are negated, controlled, made conditional and interspersed with epistemic, colonialist, ableist and classed inequalities. If we read abortion trail activism against the contentions of reproductive justice without conceptualizing abortion trail activism as reflective of a political project, there is a risk of artificially separating abortion trail activism from reproductive justice due to the former's explicit focus on abortion. By interpreting abortion trail activism as prefigurative politics – and thereby recognizing abortion trail activists' efforts to lessen the financial burden of abortion, for example, as intended to address uneven reproductive economies – it is possible to avoid the separation of this specific form of activist work from the deeper politics of reproductive justice.

Third, and finally, prefiguration also helps connect the commitments identified in the preceding chapters as a consistent feature of abortion trail activism with an overarching political praxis. By conceiving of abortion trail activism as a prefigurative politics, we can critically engage with what futures this form of political action is attempting to prefigure. Based on the accounts of activists, we can see a will to rework abortion as accessible through an infrastructure of care that sees abortion as ontological and non-normative. There is an active effort to disrupt the relations of power and knowledge that limit access. The aspiration is fundamentally to reconstructive abortion access as unconditional and the experience of abortion care as characterized by support, facilitation and respect. Prefiguration provides us with a political vocabulary to discuss actions that are inspired by these goals. This vocabulary is important not just because it allows us to engage with abortion trail activism analytically, as a mode of politics, rather than descriptively. It is also important because it addresses the problem raised by one organizer in an abortion trail group (which they addressed as a practical support network) in the United States – how can we talk about something that is just about human existence? The essential point here is that, through prefiguration, it is possible to interrogate the political intent of actions that first appear as acts of goodwill.

Having proposed a working interpretation of abortion trail activism beyond description of specific organizations, I want to now put this interpretation to work. Building on the argument that abortion trails and abortion trail activism constitute a distinguishable political practice, I want to reflect on what distinguishing abortion trail activism adds to our understanding of the contestations within pro-choice abortion politics. In the remaining chapters, I argue that we can use abortion trails as an analytic mechanism to make visible a central tension within the pro-choice abortion project between allowing abortion trails to be persistent and seeking the integration of abortion trail within a sanctioned, regulated abortion care architecture. As part of this discussion – and again demonstrating the usefulness of trails as a framework – the chapters consider the role of framings of abortion trails in orientating the pro-choice abortion project towards formalization, what narrative foreclosures the framings of trails produce and the problems that arise when abortion trails are 'formalized'.

4

Abortion trails and the Narrative of Pro-Choice

Introduction

The preceding three chapters provide an image of abortion trail activism as a species of abortion politics characterized by an orientation towards accessibility, a commitment feminist ethics of care and engagement in prefigurative action. The discussions in these chapters enable us to connect the different activists, activisms and mobilizations in diverse jurisdictions at a range of time-points as part of a shared political praxis. This intervention enables us to move from the descriptive to the discursive – by positioning diverse actors as manifestations of a specifiable political ideology it is possible to engage with the logics of this political praxis.

In the book's Introduction I suggested the benefits of trails as analytic devices that foreground contradictions within established ways of thinking. This will be the focus of the remainder of this book. In this and the following chapter, I want to examine the differing framings of abortion trails and how these shape the direction of pro-choice abortion politics. I am particularly interested in using abortion trails to highlight the contestations over moving towards a finished or built formal architecture of abortion access and care (as a goal of abortion politics) as well as the fundamental flaws with the notion of a finished/built architecture. Working along similar themes, and consistent with the introductory chapter's reflection on trails, the reflections in these chapters will unpack the varying readings of abortion trails and abortion trail activism.

I want to demonstrate the tensions within abortion politics that *framings* of abortion trails and abortion trail work raise in relation to the intents of pro-choice abortion politics. This discussion is distinct from the tensions that the *work* of abortion trail activists highlight. It returns to the larger recognition of trails nebulousness and how differing perspectives of trails – as liberation, for example, or danger – connect to and produce socio-political discourses. Here I further the argument that, rather than move towards categorizing different forms of abortion trail work, we should use the nebulousness of abortion trails as an analytic opening. Through engaging with framings of abortion trails, I contend that we can read the contesting perspectives on what the intent of abortion politics is or should be.

Abortion trails and the narratives of pro-choice

Trails are effervescent and ultimately ambiguous. The introductory chapter identified some potential readings of trails – as lines of desire, spatialized memories, urban resistance and *panya* – each of which both offered a different interpretation of what a trail is and illustrated the complexities of trails. A trail can be emancipatory, liberating and enterprising; it can also be demanded, governed and oppressive. It blends history and futurity, the planned and the providential, and function and conservation. Comparing the different presentations of trails – as security threats (*panya*, county lines) or enacted mobile resistance (lines of desire) – as well as critical analysis of trails as the site of queer exclusions or persistent colonialist land-occupation is not simply interesting intellectually. It draws attention to what Clare Hemmings (2005, 2011, 2018) discusses as narrative politics. Hemmings' interventions echo those articulated by decolonial studies – particularly the work of Vazquéz (2009) on the erosive effect of Westernized histories of progress and modernity on colonized societies and cultures. Centrally, these bodies of knowledge consider how storytelling and the establishment of accepted narratives reinforce the positioning of the trajectories of the Global North as typifying, or indeed the fundamental representation of, progress.

Hemmings' argument is that narratives which present feminist history as linear progression and development over waves, generations or time periods raise problems both in terms of appreciating the richness and complexity of feminist politics within and outside the Global North/West and risk-emboldening binary interpretations of feminism. These binary interpretations include the idea that feminism has become meaningful (for those at the peripheries) or meaningless (for those who do not meet the supposed standards of 'diversity politics'). Furthermore, the presentation of recent feminist history as progress or development from discrimination to liberation can reinforce colonialist epistemic politics which either erases or dismisses the Global South's history. Again, the effects of this are complex and range from promoting a vernacularization of Global North feminism – its transport to and translation into the discourses of the Global South – as the best path to gender development to the conflation of all feminist politics – including those generated by feminist activists in the Global South – as a continuation of colonialism.

Hemmings' stated aim is to understand how narrative politics reinforce a particular story about feminism where specific knowledges and practices are treated as axiomatic or 'common sense' (Hemmings, 2005). The effect of this intervention is to position narrative framings as analytic devices for querying feminist theory. The focus of her analysis is a bounded narrative – feminist theory – communicated through academic writing and teaching. However, and significantly for the study of subjects which lack this bounded character, narrative presentations can also offer ample analytic possibilities. The Introduction to this book already indicates how examination of the narratives and knowledges attached to more effervescent objects – trails – can act as an entry to a larger reflection about what shapes 'common sense' or established framings of these objects.

The discussion of trails also indicated how framings of objects which are being continuously remade and remain under construction result in narrative foreclosures as the spirit of an ultimately ambivalent assemblage is connected to distinct interpretations. This manifests in the examples of the *panya* and *chemins de désir* which, whether being addressed as dangerous or emancipatory, are locked into a narrative of their nature. Furthermore, and critically, these framings are not always explicitly stated but articulated through how activities on or within *panya*/lines of desire are described. The description of those who use *panya* as engaged in illicit activities implicitly frames this trail as dangerous. More importantly, policies narratives and agendas which intersect with trails – how best to design urban space, for instance, or how to manage cross-border trading routes – emerge from and are shaped by these framings.

Carse and Kneas (2019) offer an important example of how planning narratives and agendas are reinforced through the treatment of objects, infrastructures or plans as 'unbuilt' or 'unfinished'. For these authors, the labels unbuilt or unfinished operate dialectally relative to the stories we tell about policy intents and trajectories. Through presenting something as stalled, intents emerge as 'a linear succession of phases or stages oriented toward meeting pre-defined objectives' (Carse and Kneas, 2019: 11). These comments are relevant to abortion trails as they demonstrate how framings of one assemblage – a thing, object, infrastructure or plan – meaningfully shape the real or imagined goals of the discourse it intersects with. Literature on abortion and reproductive justice politics has noted the effects of narratives of the aspiration of activists on imaginings of the intent of political projects which they use as a comparative referent. For example, writing on reproductive justice narratives in the US context, Thomsen (2015) argues that these construct particular imaginings of reproductive rights through emphasizing reproductive justice as markedly different. My aim here is not to repeat Thomsen's discussion of reproductive justice narratives of reproductive rights; rather, I want to explore the narratives produced by framings of abortion trails and the effects of this on the pro-choice political project. This includes framings which position abortion trails as legally outside, as lifelines and as a shadow infrastructure. These framings are articulated both through descriptions of abortion trails and the work of abortion trail activists of what trails offer.

According to Thomsen, reproductive justice's self-articulation as a more capacious understanding of histories of reproductive violence, forms of reproductive violence, and mechanisms for addressing reproductive violence cemented a perspective on reproductive rights as a White feminist politics almost wholly concerned with abortion rights, privacy and choice. While the aspiration to expand justice beyond abortion rights is a positive one, grounded in the experience of marginalized communities, Thomsen contends that the consistent emphasis on addressing more than abortion marginalizes the pursuit of abortion access within the panoply of reproductive justice political objectives. The work to differentiate justice from rights, Thomsen suggests, partly obscures the importance of addressing the significant barriers to abortion rights facing communities who have experienced multiple forms of reproductive harms. The narrative of reproductive justice as an intentional expansive politics of and against reproductive harms as opposed to reproductive rights as a narrow politics of pro-choice abortion rights, Thomsen's critique implies, undermines the objective of reproductive justice to avoid stratifying reproductive injustices. Reproductive justice can, through its self-articulation as a corrective to the prioritization of abortion rights above, for example, forced sterilization, obstetric violence, coerced abortion or child removal, side-line abortion within conversations of reproductive autonomy.

In terms of abortion trails, the key point to draw here relates to the political effect of narratives and how this can work at cross purposes to the aspirations of those supporting political mobilizations. Reproductive justice works expansively on itself, distinguishing its own politics from those of pro-choice reproductive rights which are positioned as narrow. However, in framing reproductive rights as narrative, reproductive justice narrows the space for pro-choice reproductive rights conversations within the terrain of reproductive justice. What I want to argue here and in the following chapter is that abortion trails experience a similar narrative problem. However, in this case the referent is not reproductive rights nor reproductive justice but a formal,

State-controlled, medical architecture. Abortion trails are framed as offering something that States do not offer or actively oppose. While this framing is embedded within a celebration of abortion trails – as a more feminist, caring form of accessing abortion – it is also woven into a narrative complaint about State failures. This has a political effect on the pro-choice movement, which is caught between pursuing greater recognition of the value of abortion trails as trails and requesting the positive attributes of trails to be absorbed by or integrated into a formalized institutional architecture.

This chapter will outline how framings constitute trails as separate from a formalized State architecture. I consider three framings of abortion trails – as legally outside, as a lifeline and as a shadow infrastructure. I will pay attention to how these narrative constitutions, at turns, celebrate and problematize abortion trails. I will also note how they do not necessarily reflect the reality of abortion trails, particularly where they collapse abortion trails into a single set of actors or disconnect it from actors within State-managed or formal health institutions (e.g. public health centres, pharmacists, health care providers) entirely. That said, despite the celebratory tones of some abortion trail narratives, which position them as enactments of feminist ethics of care (see Chapters 2 and 3; McReynolds-Perez et al., 2023; Duffy, Freeman and Castañeda, 2023), framings of abortion trails also present their existence as indicative of a problematic attitude to and exclusion of essential reproductive health support by the State. Abortion trails are presented, at times, as demonstrative of uncare or the absence of abortion care, as dangerous, and as used due to a lack of safe access routes (see Erdman, Jelinska and Yanow, 2018 for critiques). In the next chapter, I argue that these framings have a political effect, orientating pro-choice abortion progress towards reducing the negative aspects of abortion trails through formalization and regulation. The problem with this narrative politics is that it forecloses the ambiguity and potential creativity of abortion trails and positions them as transgressive (Nandagiri and Pizzarossa, 2023) as opposed to generative to new modes of abortion access and care. More directly, it results in approaches to liberalizing abortion that do not challenge inequalities in access. To illustrate this latter point I use the examples of the Republic of Ireland and Colombia.

Framings of abortion trails

Abortion trails as legally outside

Legal outsideness is a dominant theme across representations and constructions of abortion trails in public and academic articulations as well as activist conversations. Writing on the Jane Collective in the United States (Kaplan, 2019; O'Donnell, 2017) on abortion pill distribution networks in the European context (e.g. in relation to Ireland, Poland and Malta; Calkin, 2023; Chełstowska and Ignaciuk, 2023), and on routes to abortion in some parts of Latin American and the Caribbean (Singer, 2019; Freeman and Rodriguez, 2023) are exemplary of how abortion trails are positioned within narratives of legality and the law. Within this framing includes the presentation of abortion trails as *outside* the law and as *illegal*. Recognition of outsideness *and* illegality is important in this instance. Sociological interpretations of the law as a juridical technology of power – particularly the work of Foucault (2012) – illegality signifies the existence of an identifiable manifestation of State sovereignty or mechanism of control. Writing on the introduction of migration legislation in the United States, scholars such as Ackerman (2014) and Ngai (2004) address illegality as a discursive formation that emerges in tandem with bordered forms of Statehood and practices of sovereignty.

Research on abortion politics and law (Bloomer, Pierson and Estrada, 2018; Gavigan, 1984) delineates between abortion trails as outside legal frameworks and abortion trails as constructed as illegal through juridical mechanisms (i.e. laws prohibiting abortion trails or technologies for directly limiting their operation). The former framing is more capacious and recognizes that abortion trails are assemblages which cut through spaces whether there is no legal framework or where the law does not restrict their use for the purposes of accessing abortion. The presentation of abortion trails as outside the law is most pronounced in writing on abortion travel and self-managed abortion using medications. Within this body of work, abortion trails work across a liminal position, on the peripheries of what is subject to regulation or what is lawful. Abortion trails between the island of Ireland and England before the period 2018–20 which saw the liberalization of abortion access in the Republic (in 2018) and the decriminalization of abortion in Northern Ireland (in 2020; Bloomer and Campbell, 2022). Travelling extrajudicially for abortion care, while contested in the Republic of Ireland in the early 1990s (De Londras and Enright, 2018; Gilmartin and White, 2011) and always undertaken at personal cost, was never prohibited entirely along a continuum of legality/illegality.

These abortion trails – which still exist and are used regularly by those whose needs fall outside the boundaries of what is legally permissible or who live in Northern Ireland, where services have not been commissioned fully by the Northern Irish Health Services – were and are not strictly speaking illegal. Yet the trails, their collective remaking through regular abortion travel and the repair work of abortion trail activists, were and are contemporaneously (re)constituted by side-along borders established by a range of legislative and regulatory instruments. Key among these was the regulation prohibiting abortion access on the island of Ireland, except in extreme circumstances. However, other co-existent instruments also shaped and constituted the trails, including the right to travel across borders, the permissibility of providing information about where and how to access services and the right to access health care as a non-resident. Abortion trails therefore are formed as outside a range of different regulatory instruments, even if not prohibited directly or strictly speaking illegal.

Abortion trails which involve the movement of abortion medicines or purchase of abortion medicines from pharmacies (Calkin and Freeman, 2019; Calkin, 2023) are similarly presented as legally outside and, at times, illegal. Assis (2020) documents the status of these abortion trails in the context of Brazil and Argentina. Subsequent to the discovery that the medication misoprostol could be used safely as an abortifacient by feminist activists in Brazil in the 1980s, regulations on medication abortion and self-managed abortion have been introduced and altered in both jurisdictions, creating abortion trails that cut across the boundaries of legality and illegality. At times, as Assis notes, misoprostol was not legally governed as an abortion medication. As such the abortion trail fell outside the law. Neither was it fully condoned as a technology for self-managed medication abortion. Like in other jurisdictions, there were other regulations against abortion and the sale of medications for the purposes of abortion that restricted abortion trails which involved purchasing medicines from pharmacies.

Considering the presentation of abortion trails as legally outside is useful as it guides us towards a more nuanced conversation about the *intent* of legal instruments or discursive processes of rendering abortion trails as governable terrain (Foucault, 2019). Resonating with Carse and Kneas' (2019) use of narratives of 'unfinished' or 'incomplete' plans to interrogate the intents of planners, reflecting on the framing of abortion trails as legally outside, a capacious framing including being illegal and being outside the territory of existing legislation or legal instruments, provides an opening to consider the objectives of legal interventions. What emerges from evidence on abortion trails which involve travel to clinics and those which involve distribution or purchase of abortion medicines or other abortifacients is an imagining of trails as shaped by legal instruments but neither always subject to nor prohibited by legal instruments of a sovereign (state) actor. Singer (2019) describes these trails as an 'alegal' exercise as 'it takes place outside of the legal systems and is commonly understood to be illegal, but is not expressly forbidden in the law' (Singer, 2019: 168).

This insight raises the question as to under what conditions, or for what reason, are abortion trails rendered governable or subjected to juridical restrictions? The most obvious answer to this is to restrict access to abortions. However, this answer is not wholly convincing given the persistence, and indeed acceptance, of abortion trails is both restrictive and liberal regimes. While in certain jurisdictions – particular areas in the United States following the Supreme Court's overturning of *Roe v Wade* through the *Dobbs v Jackson Women's Health Centre* – abortion trails have been subjected to intensive interventions to reduce abortion access, this is arguably an exceptional rather than a conventional formulation of the relationship between abortion trails and the law. A more commonly observed dynamic between abortion trails and governance is the reconstitution of abortion trails as the borders between legal abortion provision and possible forms of abortion provision and access change. Side (2021) considers this in her discussion of how abortion laws and abortion technologies introduce sites of mobility and fixity. Trails emerge and change as new sites of regulation and objects of legal intervention are inscribed on the ontological, and immutable, reality that abortion will ultimately outlast any form of legal intervention, even if it means abortion seekers absorb a substantial risk to life or personal burden. They are constituted, by the introduction of governing technologies such as abortion laws or regulations on medicine use, as legally outside not as part of a project of restricting abortion access but of restricting particular forms of abortion access.

Using the narrative positioning of abortion trails as legally outside offers an opening to reflect on the effect of this framing on the orientation of the pro-choice movement. As already discussed in earlier chapters, the relationship between abortion trails and legal instruments directs the mobilizations of activists, who work to repair and maintain abortion trails, to make abortion more accessible and to prefigure a practice of abortion consistent with a feminist ethic of care. Again, the status of abortion trails as legally outside does not just produce forms of activism that address the effects of legal/illegal bordering. It also results in distinguishable political mobilizations towards addressing the effects of co-existent legal instruments or absences in legal frameworks designed to permit abortion access. The work of abortion trail activists who predominantly work with migrant populations – such as abortion trail activists working with migrants and asylum seekers in the

Netherlands and Ireland – exemplifies how trail *work* is shaped by legal outsideness.

How the existence of legally outside abortion trails which, while unsanctioned, are neither necessarily nor always illegal, shapes pro-choice activism is more complex. There are visible examples of where abortion trails have expanded the concerns of the pro-choice movement to include the safety and availability of abortion technologies. Abortion medications are the clearest representation of this, as documented in work on the movement of abortion pills (including enhancing their accessibility) and calls for support for self-managed abortion from the periphery to the centre of pro-choice advocacy (Calkin, 2023; Berro Pizzarossa and Nandagiri, 2021).

At the same time, these shifts in abortion trails have not been translated into a single or unified aim across pro-choice politics globally. The intent – or 'ask' – of pro-choice actors in response to the emergence of medication abortion and accompaniment practices varies. Nandagiri and Berro Pizzarossa (2021, 2023) highlight this, describing self-managed abortion as subject to a 'cacophony' of legal instruments and noting that the response to abortion pill or self-managed abortion trails by pro-choice movements had created new sites of transgression as self-management has been constituted through schemas of acceptable medical practices. This is a very different interpretation of the effect of abortion trails than that alluded to by Singer (2019) who argues that 'alegal' trails challenge and push pro-choice actors beyond requesting reform from the State, 'seizing abortion rights, rather than seeking to implement them through legalistic channels' (Singer, 2019: 168).

The intent of pro-choice politics remains, in Nandagiri and Berro Pizzarossa's (2023) argument, establishing a legalistic channel for abortion access. The difference is that this channel can, in some circumstances, include self-management and medication abortion. These authors' intervention, particularly on the new sites of transgression created by the aspiration to address illegality, is important as it invites us to reflect on whether this aspiration will have positive effects. The key question here is whether being legally outside or unsanctioned is inherently problematic. Critically engaging with the framing of abortion trails as legally outside shows that a straightforward interpretation of abortion trails as illegal entities does not fully capture either the function or essence of the trails. Furthermore, it opens up important questions regarding the intentions of pro-choice politics and the effects of pursuing these intentions (e.g. the creation of new modes of transgression).

Abortion trails as a 'lifeline'

The second framing of abortion trails present within commentaries is as a 'lifeline'. This interpretation is particularly pronounced in restrictive regimes, where abortion access is extremely limited or expressly prohibited by legal frameworks. A recent iteration of the lifeline framing emerged in the US context, following the Supreme Court's 2022 decision on *Dobbs v Jackson Women's Health Organisation*, which overturned the 1973 *Roe v Wade* judgement. *Roe* had acted as a de facto national protection of the right to abortion. In its absence, State-level legislatures can now introduce legislation that criminalizes provision of abortion, accessing abortion within State and/or acts as a near-total abortion ban (e.g. prohibiting abortion beyond six-weeks' gestation or except in extreme case, where there is an immediate risk to life). Some States have, following *Dobbs*, expanded existing restrictions designed to target abortion providers (TRAP laws) such as regulations on what health care should be financed through the US's public health insurance programme (Medicaid) or the need for providing facilities to be particular distances from other amenities. Abortion-seeking has also become subject to more extensive surveillance and deterrence. Measures include the introduction of financial inducements to encourage members of the public to report suspected illegal abortions ('bounty hunting') and enabling law enforcement to use data from period-tracking applications on personal devices in criminal investigations.

There is a temptation to position *Dobbs* as a drastic reversal of a status quo where abortion was generally accessible. However, abortion providers and reproductive rights and justice groups had reported the steady encroachments of abortion access, despite *Roe*, prior to *Dobbs*. TRAP laws, limitations on Medicaid, compulsory 'reflection' or waiting times between consultations with abortion providers and the closure of clinics due to underfunding had undermined access long before the 2022 Supreme Court judgement. Recognizing the persistent attempts to disrupt access through regulatory mechanisms after *Roe* and prior to *Dobbs* is important not just to draw attention to the fact that abortion trails have continuously operated in the United States but that, in the United States, they have operated within a context where abortion access has been repeatedly challenged.

This has contributed to a popular framing of abortion trails as 'lifelines', used in extreme circumstances, where means of accessing abortion are being or have been systematically eroded. Activists, including some interviewed during the research underpinning this book, also project an image of abortion trails as 'lifelines'. This includes activists supporting physical trails (e.g. cross-border routes, logistical support networks), activists involved in supporting both access to and the use of abortion pills and activists providing information and financial support. Abortion trails were presented in interviews as enabling abortion access within contexts where abortion was criminalized and the alternative, as alluded to in the account for an activist below, was unsafe abortion. Here the respondent outlines how they positioned abortion trail activists as supporting 'lifelines' within the African context, where abortion is frequently both criminalized and stigmatized. For the respondent below, starting with personal stories was a particularly effective way of disrupting the attitudes of conservative families, many of whom, according to this activist, also live in poverty:

'What if it was your daughter? You wake her up and then she's dead, what would you choose? What would you wish for? Would you wish her like she would have died? Or you would have wished she would have talked to you and then you would have forged the way forward?'

The abortion cases that happen among young girls and it's because they are coming from poverty families, families with very, very conservative parents, very hard, very . . . You cannot talk to them, you know? So what happens if the child chooses another way? Like she chooses another option and then in the end she might get problems. And that's when the parents now realise that, 'Okay, other than losing my child, who would have talked to me? Who would have found another way than dying?' So, we bring the whole abortion. We bring all the stories on the death of unsafe abortion. We bring all those cases and then we tell them that at least every day, fourteen women die every day due to unsafe abortion in [country]. So, we are there to protect women. 'Cause, even if you deny that abortion is illegal, people are still accessing the service, you know? And they are accessing unsafely. So, bring it. And then that's when people have a mind change. (Abortion activist, Africa)

Like the 'legally outside' framing, the 'lifelines' presentation of abortion trails underscores the ontological and immutable character of abortion care. At the same time, it has been critiqued by scholars for conveying an image of abortion trails as used out of desperation and, by implication, unsafe (Erdman, Jelinska and Yanow, 2018). This is reflected in the comments from the interviewee cited above. In this activists' account, conversations of abortion trails are closely connected with individual desperation and the concomitant necessity of using potentially fatal modes of care.

Such a positioning reinforces problematic representations of abortion trail activism, which as noted in previous chapters, are part of a prefigurative politics of constructing modes of abortion care that resonate more closely with feminist ethics of care in the present moment. While abortion trails can act as lifelines to those who are unable to access abortion through other means, presenting them only or mainly as a 'lifeline' both obscures the resistant and prefigurative aims of activists. The 'abortion trails as lifelines' also suggests that they are brought into existence as an extraordinary mechanism. As indicated by the activist above, drawing on spectacular, extraordinary harms can be useful to initiating conversations about the everyday nature of abortion-seeking. At the same time, there is a risk here of depicting abortion itself as a spectacular, rather than a quotidian or ontological, reproductive experience.

The amplification of 'lifelines' in the context of intensive regulation or criminalization – whether by legal mechanisms, social stigma or unwillingness to provide abortion care by health professionals – is thus problematic. Abortion trails are discursively constituted through the lifelines narrative as resulting from the absence of a more formal pathway. The implication of the 'lifelines' image is that it would not be used if a means of legal, socially acceptable mode accessing abortion in clinical settings existed. Yet this is not consistent with either the reality of abortion trail usage or the position of all abortion trail activists. While there is a recognition that abortion trails are a 'lifeline' for those in contexts where accessibility is limited, there is an equal recognition that abortion trails are used in circumstances where there are officially sanctioned abortion pathways in safe settings. Abortion trails in these contexts act as 'lifelines' not because abortion is not available but because an alternative experience of care is desired or required. The most obvious example of this is the use of pharmaceutical abortion trails within countries like England and Wales, where there are abortion clinics and an established legal framework, by people who need or wish to have an abortion at home.

Abortion trails as a shadow infrastructure

The framings above are more well established in public consciousness and popular representations of abortion trails and certainly those emanating from English-speaking contexts. However, there is a further framing of abortion trails that I want to draw attention to – abortion trails as shadow infrastructures. This framing presents abortion trails as a dynamic assemblage addressing ontological needs which are either unmet or neglected by the State. Shadow infrastructures, as I outline in this section, are tonally different to legal outsideness or lifelines as they highlight and at points celebrate abortion trails as agile and dynamic infrastructures that embrace the possibility for care provision to be promiscuous or offered by strangers (Chatzidakis et al, 2020).

Scholars based in science and technology studies (STS), sociology of health and political and human geography have used infrastructures as an analytic device for foregrounding the material, mundane, technical but ultimately political, relational and social architectures that shape, facilitate and sustain care. As Danholt and Langstrup (2012) summarize 'infrastructures of care are the more or less embedded "tracks" on which care may "run", shaping and being shaped by actors and settings along the way' (pg. 514). Conceptually, the infrastructural turn (Alam and Houston, 2020) brings together writing on how networks of actors, including human and non-human objects and things, produce social order, subjecthood and social functioning (Latour, 2007) with discussions of materiality and the role of practices and objects in shaping experience. The starting point for infrastructural analysis is that infrastructures exist but are neither inert nor innate; rather they are dynamic, produced discursively and emergent. The agility and relationality of infrastructures also means that there is no master epistemology or framework directing their operations; they are constantly being reorganized and reworked. Danholt and Langstrup (2012) provide a further useful explanation of infrastructural analysis's key points in the following text:

> Infrastructures are [. . .] contingent, social and historical constructs. They have a point of origin, and have undergone transformations over time owing to numerous contingent processes and negotiations. They are heterogeneous, since no single overarching logic or principle has formed them, and they are constructed and function as they do thanks to a heterogeneous conglomeration of political, technical, social, economic, historical, practical and other reasons. (Danholt and Langstrup, 2012: 517)

An important contribution of infrastructural analysis is that it underlines the potential role of individuals in reforming and maintaining infrastructures and, as a consequence, the entanglement of infrastructures with power relations between subjects. This analytic position emphasizes the ambiguity and fluidity of infrastructures. Furthermore, infrastructural analysis is very clear on the immanence of infrastructures. The things, relationships and practices that make up and are made up by infrastructures are not created out of nothing; we become aware of them depending on our positionality (consider for example how we encounter a railway when we need to travel). They are therefore, 'never simply there or not there, but partially and potentially existing and emergent' (Danholt and Langstrup, 2012: 518).

The purpose of infrastructural analysis is to enrich the conversation regarding the things, practices and perceptions that surround and run through everyday interactions so that we recognize the historic, political, economic and social contingencies of these interactions. This allows us to direct our critiques at, on the one hand, the disciplinary and regulatory character of infrastructures and, on the other, the potential for social and discursive disruption infrastructures present. Infrastructures are sites of contestation. Moreover, writing on infrastructures of care argues that, while the organization of infrastructures in the present moment has an origin, as care is an ontological species activity (Tronto and Fisher, 1990), we cannot approach infrastructural care analysis from the position that there was no infrastructure, or components that constitute an infrastructure, before the present moment. Mesman (2011) argues that, if we accept this, we need to undertake *exnovation*, a term which according to Mesman,

> refers to the attempt to foreground what is already present – though hidden – in specific practices, to render explicit what is implicit in them. Where innovation can be defined as 'to make something new', exnovation pays attention to what is already in place and challenges the dominant trend to discard existing practices [. . .] A focus on exnovation allows us to bring to light implicit matters of actual practice and to develop a fresh perspective on the ingenuity of the professional and the specific structure of their practices. (Mesman, 2011: 5)

Echoing this call to interrogate the 'present but hidden' infrastructures of care, Power et al. (2022) have explored 'shadow' care infrastructures in post-welfare regimes. Like Mesman, the starting point for Power et al.'s analysis is that, while infrastructural arrangements and practices may be limited and problematic, they are an immutable part of human relationalities. It thus follows that, in circumstances where the care infrastructures of the State, the object of Power et al.'s analysis, fall short, shadow care infrastructures will fill residual gaps. This framing is consistent with infrastructural research in geography which looks at 'repair and maintenance' work, as well as feminist writing on care which stresses that, due to the ontological nature of care and caring relations, gaps in care infrastructures are not spaces of absent carelessness (which is not possible) but spaces which generate new forms or alternative forms of care (Puig de la Bellacasa, 2017).

Power et al. call for a more considered attentiveness to shadow care infrastructures both to acknowledge their existence and to subject their practices, internal dynamics and logics to greater scrutiny. As these authors explain:

> When light is shone on phenomena [. . .] certain features are foregrounded, while others fall into the shadows, unseen or appearing differently to how they might if light were directed toward them. [. . .] Shadow care infrastructures plays with this idea to purposefully draw focus to spaces, practices and resources that enable survival within post-welfare cities and exist both withing and between dominant political and research lenses. Thinking with shadows is to ask: 'what is there that is not readily seen or acknowledged?' (Power et al., 2022: 1172)

Analysis of shadow care infrastructures encourages us to move beyond erasing or overlooking the complex networks of practices and actors that exist within and between more recognizable or 'official' infrastructures of care. This call is important not just because it again reminds us that infrastructures of care are not limited to established architectures of the State, for example, but also, by presenting these shadow infrastructures as enabling 'survival', foregrounds the dynamism and potentially resistant qualities of these infrastructures. Shadow infrastructures of care, within Power et al.'s analysis of post-welfare regimes in the UK, are shaped by both the absence of State welfare and the discursive orientation of State infrastructures of care towards 'un-care'. The term refers to the practices, mechanisms and networks can exist and operate beyond a formal architecture – in Power et al.'s research this is mainly the formal welfare-State infrastructure.

Shadow infrastructure is not a term used in writing about abortion trails or by abortion trail activists directly. There are some potential proxies for 'shadows' – backstreet, underground or hidden, for example – but, unlike 'lifelines' or legal outsideness, 'shadow infrastructure' is not obviously part of abortion trail narratives or public discourse. However, the language used by activists and their allies as well as scholarship on this species of activism to describe abortion trails and the work of activists on them resonates strongly with this framing. For example, activists from a US-based network for people seeking later-gestation abortions interviewed as part of the research underpinning this book, presented their interventions as supporting care needs that fall outside existing architectures of health care. As a co-ordinator explains in the interview quote below:

> In terms of accessibility to this care, if you think about early-stage abortions, they are much more easy to get usually, there are less barriers to get to that care, it's less expensive. Much, much less expensive, in the US especially. Later abortions can be up to tens of thousands of dollars. And so, that on top of the cost of travelling long distances. It seemed to make sense to support those people who are experiencing a lot more burdens getting to their care. (Abortion activist, US2)

Writing on and by accompaniment networks, including practical support or abortion travel groups and information hotlines, also frames abortion trails as an infrastructure that works around and supports the needs that fall outside a formal infrastructure of abortion care. Information hotlines, for example, offer guidance on the embodied experience of taking abortion pills (such as pain levels to expect and when to seek care). Many also offer emotional support, which they argue is not offered within the existing infrastructures of abortion care (Larrea et al., 2021; Veldhuis, Sánchez-Ramírez and Darney, 2022b).

What is interesting about the framing of abortion trails as a shadow infrastructure is that it does not fit well with assumptions about trails more generally, particularly the interpretation of trails as inherently unstructured. The 'lifelines' and 'legally outside' framings resonate much more strongly with an imagining of trails as ad hoc or less organized. However, as noted in the book's Introduction, the construction of trails as haphazard, disorganized or even organic obscures the fact that trails are frequently closely managed and encompass a range of practices and relationships which maintain and refine their operations. Abortion trails as shadow infrastructures therefore have important analytic value, not only as a means of reflecting on how narrative framings of abortion trails impact the narratives and intents of the pro-choice project but also as a mechanism for foregrounding the divergences between narratives of the essence of abortion trails. Unlike lifelines or legal outsideness, 'shadow infrastructures' is not directly stated and does not connect abortion trails to a rough-and-ready aesthetic. This framing becomes visible through the accounts of activists on the location of their work – in the shadows, gaps and spaces outside a formal assemblage of practices and things – and positions abortion trails as an organized, refined mechanism defined by functionality.

At the same time, like the other framings, examination of this positioning of abortion trails raises important questions for pro-choice narratives. Power et al (2022) do not advocate appreciating shadow infrastructures uncritically. On the contrary, they underline the need to scrutinize shadow infrastructures to avoid neglecting their ambivalent, and thus the potentially problematic, internal politics. Like all care infrastructures, and care itself, shadow care infrastructures are formed within, through and in relation to discursive power relations, subjectivities and subject-positions which are inequitable and restrictive. These inequalities are reproduced through subject relations and practices, and are entangled with shadow care infrastructures. What emerges within and through the shadows may indeed, as Puig de la Bellacasa indicates, generate new, resistant forms of care. However, it may also reinforce inequities and discursive problematics.

Sociological theory has consistently stressed the very real possibility for marginalized actors, including those imbricated in shadow care infrastructures, to reproduce uneven subjectivities and subject-positions. This argument is central to Bev Skeggs' (1997) arguments on the formation of gendered subjectivities through matrices of classed inequalities within working-class communities. Skeggs' analysis, developed through ethnographic analysis of working-class women in Northern England, underscores the fact that a life on the margins or outside is not unconstrained by or unencumbered with classed expectations or regulations. Research on political geography and activism through infrastructures outside the State has also indicated the need to look closely at these informal infrastructures before assuming their resistant political intentions or character. Kamal (2023), for example, theorizes such infrastructures as 'mundane activism' which repairs, maintains and fills gaps within and between formal infrastructures but does not seek to disrupt the discursive or political terrain.

Critical engagement with the politics of infrastructures of care, including those generated by and within the 'shadows', is essential, according to Power et al. (2022). Such critical engagement 'can foreground the unevenness of systems that support care practices, raising awareness of how deprivation is variously reinforced or overcome through the way care infrastructures come together' (pp 1175). It also avoids the, arguably romantic, presumption of the benevolence or positive additionality of shadow infrastructures of care and ensures we accept that such networks are not always 'well resourced, coherent or work well' (pp 1176). Interrogating shadow infrastructures of care directly, according to these authors, sustains a consistent scrutiny of 'the interests that are selectively encoded into infrastructures and that differentially shape access and use' (pp. 1175) as well as 'who is included and excluded and why' (pp 1178).

Returning to the question of abortion trail narrative framing, these comments are important. They foreground both the necessity of querying what gaps or absences are underscored by activists in their articulations of abortion trails and the possibility of, once again, using framings of abortion trails to draw attention to the complexities of pro-choice politics. What is interesting about the positioning of abortion trails as a shadow infrastructure is its formative effects, by comparison, on imaginings of the formal or official infrastructure. By addressing abortion trails as the networks and practices that exist within the 'shadows', this framing implicitly produces an image of a more formal counterpart which addresses a finite array of abortion care needs and abortion-seeking communities. This effect is visible in how activists position their work as directed at the points where already-marginalized groups access, or rather fail to access, abortion care.

Additionally, this framing raises questions in relation to the pro-choice project, particularly whether the intent should be expanding formal infrastructures to address needs currently addressed in the shadows or to engage in dialogue with and learn from the shadows. The latter intent is more complex and requires not just an acceptance that not all needs can be met by a formal infrastructure but also a commitment to treating abortion trails as spaces where new requirements and ways of accessing and providing care emerge. At the same time, this respect for the generative possibilities of shadow infrastructures and abortion trails needs to be counterweighted with the uncritical valorization that Power et al. (2022) recognize – spaces of alterity are ambiguous and as such their benevolence cannot be assumed.

Narrating pro-choice intents through abortion trails

An entry point to this chapter was the contention that framings of specific objects or entities through reference to a different version or approach can become part of a narrative politics which produces and orientates a social and political mobilization. Social theory contains numerous examples of this process, highlighted across literatures from decolonial critiques of the organizing of modernity along a linear temporality of progress through the framing of current as an advanced version of a pre-colonial timespace (Vazquéz, 2009) to Hemmings' (2005) work on the production of a feminist story. Reproductive justice and abortion debates do not exist outside this narrative politics. Understandings of the reproductive rights or pro-choice abortion rights have been formed through reproductive justice's articulation of its own difference from these projects (Thomsen, 2015). Equally, framings of trails exert a narrative influence – constituting spaces as more authentic, spiritual or less safe alternatives to formal routeways (see Introduction; Moor, 2016).

However, a central intervention of the various theoretical arguments on narrative politics is that framings always involve foreclosures or selective emphases. Frequently these are articulated through binaries or referents – civil versus uncivil, reproductive justice versus pro-choice rights, trails versus paths, for example. Yet, what narrative politics contends is that binaries do not reflect the complexity of the objects that are being framed. Nevertheless, they have a meaningful discursive affect, shaping the direction and intents of social, economic or political projects. Futurities are brought into being and suspended on present imaginings, as Berlant (2020) suggested, producing subjects intent on moving towards (or away from) particular ways of being (see also Ahmed, 2020).

Moving from this position, how can we view abortion trails? My aim here is not to repeat the arguments of Thomsen (2015) regarding the constitutive effect of articulations of reproductive justice on narratives of reproductive rights. Rather I am interested in how framings of abortion trails constitute differing understandings of the State's relationship with abortion or what a formal, State-sanctioned version of abortion access looks like. More importantly, these framings present various intents for pro-choice abortion politics to pursue. In the chapter, I purposely selected framings which are commonly found in popular discussions of abortion trails – which see them as legally outside or 'lifelines' – as well as framings which are identifiable in how activists speak about trails – as shadow infrastructures to abortion care. Each of these framings constructs an image of the State as, at turns, hostile to abortion, negligent with regards the needs of abortion seekers, or permitting abortion under limited circumstances but not in ways that meaningfully allow for barrier-free access. Abortion trails are presented as operating around anti-abortion regulations, mobilizing when regulation for abortion does not exist, or addressing the gaps in official abortion infrastructures.

Crucially, what the discussion above denotes is that, echoing earlier comments about the ambiguous and non-normative nature of trails, it is perfectly possible to view aspects of abortion trails highlighted by these framings as positive. For instance, the operation of abortion trails outside legal parameters could be celebrated as illustrative of the absence of governing technologies which border abortion access and offer space for prefiguration and continuous remaking of abortion trails. Like *panya*, danger can be read into abortion trails but so too can resistance and autonomous action. This raises questions regarding the intents of pro-choice abortion politics. There is the possibility of these intents remaining attentive to autonomous abortion, outside legal constraints (Veldhuis, Sánchez-Ramírez and Darney, 2022a, 2002b). As the description of abortion trails as a shadow infrastructure and comments in Chapters 1 to 3 suggest, abortion trails are not inherently disorganized or unsafe. They may also be agile, refined and both reflect and address the needs of abortion seekers. These attributes are highlighted by activists in their articulation and framing of abortion trails.

At the same time, from a narrative politics perspective, the review above shows how framings can direct the pro-choice abortion project towards an improved formal architecture. By depicting abortion trails as extraordinary, symptomatic of anti-abortion restrictions or 'lifelines', the framings above suggest that the intent of the pro-choice abortion project should be a corrective one where the State improves the architecture of abortion and addresses the dangers of abortion trails. The next, and final, chapter will look to how these intents have gained traction. It will then consider what the interpretation of the pro-choice abortion project as a narrative of resolving the need for abortion trails or integrating the acceptable practices within abortion trails tells us about the direction and future directions of abortion politics more generally.

5

Pro-choice Abortion Projects and The Problematic Politics of Tidying Abortion Trails

Introduction

By this point, this book has established that abortion trails are diverse in their composition. Importantly, they are produced by and within specific political, legal and historical contexts. What abortion trail activists seek to repair, challenge and work through is influenced by the conditions of abortion access and contextual limitations on care or, in some spaces and places, the overt imposition of hyper-restrictive regimes of uncare. That said, it is possible, through looking across abortion trails as part of abortion history and the ontology of abortion, to see resonances in the ideologies and praxes of activists working on abortion trails. Crucially it is possible to infer that abortion trails and abortion trail activism as reflective of a distinguishable political project.

Nevertheless, if we reflect on the framings of abortion trails, it is equally possible to identify abortion trails as subject to a narrative politics where they are defined in relation to a particular referent, which I have broadly labelled the State or the formal architecture of abortion care. In the preceding chapter, by positioning abortion trails as part of a narrative politics, I sought to emphasize the analytic value of this concept beyond the descriptive value (i.e. as a means of discussing diverse mobilizations as politically resonant). Following writing on the role of narratives in feminist theory (Hemmings, 2005) and in reproductive justice research specifically (Thomsen, 2015), I contended that the framing of abortion trails had a constitutive effect on, first, what we see as the absences or problematics of the State with regard to abortion, and second, the intent of pro-choice abortion politics. By considering three framings of abortion trails, I drew attention that these were *framings*, each of which can orientate pro-choice abortion politics in various directions. For example, an interpretation of trails as *problematically* legally outside or unregulated can produce a pro-choice abortion project that aspires to render trails governable and subject it to the intervention of State-sanctioned legal instruments. Alternatively, if abortion trails legal outsideness is interpreted as enabling creativity and generative to new modes of abortion care, the resulting pro-choice political intent may be to retain this separateness.

This chapter will progress these arguments, focusing on what developments in pro-choice abortion politics suggest about the imagining of a formal or State-sanctioned abortion architecture and interpretation of abortion trails that has to date gained most traction. From this point, I want to critique the pro-choice abortion politics produced by the dominant interpretations of abortion trails. My contentions here are not based on a comparison between pro-choice politics and reproductive justice, for example, or another framework within the reproductive politics space. The referent, to build on Thomsen's phrasing, I want to use is between abortion trails as an effervescent project of accessibility, feminist care and prefiguration and a formal or State-sanctioned version of a trail. I have already introduced this argument in considering the difference between abortion trails and abortion pathways (in Chapter 1). Ultimately, I want to underline the importance of querying the value of formalizing abortion trails and what the aims of such formalization are. In doing so, I aim to open space for valuing abortion trails as an ongoing but nebulous and ambiguous praxis rather than approaching them through the descriptive lens of what means of abortion are or are not offered.

Narrative, pro-choice abortion politics and abortion trails

Narrative politics is about understanding, on the one hand, how discourses reflect, produce and form distinguishable understandings of subjects and, on the other hand, how these discourses foreclose multiple other understandings, formed and unformed. Thomsen's (2015) analysis of abortion justice and reproductive justice movements from a narrative politics perspective indicates how these reflect an understanding of rights-based arguments relating to reproductive choice as only partially addressing systemic reproductive harms. As a starting point to identifying the dominant interpretations of abortion trails within the pro-choice abortion project and how this project has been shaped by both framings of abortion trails and the resulting imagining of a formalized, State-sanctioned abortion care architecture, I want to briefly outline the present state of pro-choice abortion politics globally.

We know that 'abortion as a practice has been documented for thousands of years' (Bloomer, Pierson and Estrada, 2018: 11). Based on literature documenting the historical emergence of abortion regulations, the 1800s is arguably when the permissibility of noxious inducements to terminate a pregnancy became an active site of political contestation (Bloomer, Pierson and Estrada, 2018). Yet, neither anti-abortion law and policy nor the social stigmatization of abortion prevents abortion from happening. According to the World Health Organization's 2021 factsheet, approximately 73 million induced abortions occur globally, each year. This amounts to approximately 61 per cent of all unintended pregnancies and 29 per cent of all pregnancies.

We also know that abortion experiences are frequently, and at a global level arguably predominantly, problematic. Of the estimated 73 million induced abortions which occur each year, a significant number are risky, unsafe and directly connected with extremely poor health outcomes. The WHO estimates, based on recent figures, that 45 per cent of abortions globally are unsafe, of which 97 per cent take place in low- and middle-income countries. As the WHO's factsheet states:

More than half of all unsafe abortions, occur in Asia, most of them in south and central Asia. In Latin America and Africa, the majority (3 out of 4) of all abortions are unsafe. In Africa, nearly half of all abortions occur in the least safe circumstances. (WHO, 25 November 2021)

We know that abortion is highly contested and that it has been for some time. In the accompanying text for their 2021 World Abortion Laws Map, the Center for Reproductive Rights notes that '970 million women, representing 59% of women of reproductive age, live in countries that broadly allow abortion [. . .] 41% of women live under restrictive laws. The inability to access safe and legal abortion care impacts 700 million women worldwide' (Center for Reproductive Rights, 2021: np).

At the same time, the trend for most of the last century has been towards recognizing abortion in law. International and regional human rights declarations – not least the United Nations' Committee on the Elimination of Discrimination Against Women (CEDAW) and the African Commission on Human and Peoples' Rights, Protocol to the African Charter on Human and Peoples' Rights on the Rights of Women in Africa (Maputo Protocol) and the UN Economic and the European Committee on Social Rights (ECSR) – have sought to establish abortion as a fundamental human right that can be regulated but neither prohibited nor made prohibitively inaccessible.

Despite these instruments, there is a persistent and fluctuating trend towards retrogressive anti-abortion legislation both at a national level through maintaining, and in some instances introducing for the first time or reintroducing, laws which target abortion specifically. These anti-abortion legislative instruments range between laws prohibiting abortion completely or in all but the most extreme circumstances, where there is a risk to life, and through a refusal by members of the international community to finance services which also provide abortion. These legal frameworks target the legality of abortion access and provision of information and care by providers (Pierson and Caruana-Finkel, 2021; Krajewska, 2022). The Mexico City Regulation

– otherwise known as the Hyde Amendment or Global Gag Rule – which restricts development aid by the United States falls into this final category. Abortion has been a key target of ultraconservative social movements in countries such as Colombia (Corredor, 2021) and Poland (Krajewska, 2022).

That said, there have been significant positive inroads in the global abortion context, led by social movements, in challenging barriers to abortion. These include the successful decriminalization of abortion in Northern Ireland, Argentina and Colombia in 2019, 2021 and 2022, respectively. Decriminalization removes abortion from the risk of criminal sanctions, a move that Berer (2017) argued would ensure the following:

1. Not punishing anyone for providing safe abortion,
2. Not punishing anyone for having an abortion,
3. Not involving the police in investigating or prosecuting safe abortion provision or practise,
4. Not involving the courts in deciding whether to allow an abortion, and
5. Treating abortion like every other form of health care – that is, using best practice in service delivery, the training of providers, and the development and application of evidence-based guidelines, and applying existing law to deal with any dangerous or negligent practices. (Berer, 2017: 14)

The movement to decriminalization is intended to remove the potential negative impact of continuing to regulate abortion through the courts, criminal law and police on health professionals, who may withdraw from providing abortion for fear of criminal prosecution (Duffy et al., 2018) or on women who may fall outside the boundaries of what the law permits (Foster, 2021). Decriminalization was pursued in these three countries out of recognition, from experience and from bearing witness to how liberalization that kept abortion within the realm of criminal law had not achieved the objectives of liberalization campaigns (Bloomer and Campbell, 2022).

We also know that there are substantial issues, regardless of efforts to liberalize or decriminalize, with the overall accessibility of abortion in real terms or respect for reproductive autonomy more generally. We know that abortion remains subject to extensive material and social barriers. Macleod, Benyon-Jones and Toerien (2017) emphasize the material inequalities that limit abortion access in South Africa and Britain, detailing the need for campaigns to act according to principles of reparative justice, an additional lens to reproductive justice which they propose as a way of focusing attention on the neglected issues of accessibility. We know too that, following decriminalization, local abortion services were not commissioned in Northern Ireland until almost two years later.

We are also clearly aware of the shifts in how an abortion is accessed or performed since the expansion of pharmaceutical or medication abortions between the 1980s and 1990s has altered the global abortion landscape (Calkin, 2023). Medication abortion, using the drugs misoprostol and mifepristone taken buccally (between the gums and inside cheek), has replaced surgical abortion as the most common mode of accessing abortion. This is due to both the comparative safety of medication abortion, particularly in early pregnancy, and the resilience of medication abortion as a form of health care to interruption of services. During the first wave of Covid-19 global lockdowns and travel restrictions, medication abortion became essential to maintaining any form of abortion access for millions (Aiken et al., 2021). We know that the advancements in medication abortion potentially address, but do not fully compensate for, the challenges presented by reliance on hospital-based services. These include access to operating theatres (Stifani et al., 2022) and conscientious objection (Davis, Casey and Keogh, 2022).

The emergence of medication abortion has also emboldened the conversation about expanding abortion health provision beyond clinicians. The World Health Organization now advocates an expanded perspective on who can be an abortion health care provider and recommends the integration of community health, allied health and traditional birth attendants (Kim, Sorhaindo and Ganatra, 2020). Task-sharing initiatives have been trialled in several countries, including Sweden (Endler et al., 2020) and Uganda (Paul et al., 2014), and there is increasing recognition for the key role played by lay health intermediaries in abortion care (Berro Pizzarossa and Nandagiri, 2021).

There has been an overall shift over time towards a widening of abortion access within legally permissible and recognized pathways, co-ordinated by health services or infrastructures recognized as safe and reliable by health service actors such as the World Health Organization. These pathways do not necessarily need to be wholly or predominantly managed by clinicians. The latter point is important as it accounts for the fact that 'non-clinical' actors – including abortion seekers themselves – have become more openly addressed as abortion providers, particularly providers of medication abortions. It also accounts for the increased acceptance of abortion doulas (Campbell et al., 2021) and promotion of modelling public health abortion services around feminist accompaniment (McReynolds-Peréz et al., 2023).

There is an argument that pro-choice abortion politics is thus characterized by the steady demedicalization of abortion (Halfmann, 2012). At present, given the repeated connection of abortion with human rights, the ongoing expansion of community pathways, telemedicine/medication abortion and the adoption of accompaniment models, the demedicalization argument – constructed by Halfmann (2012) as distinct from the medicalization of abortion as a clinical concern, managed by medical professionals, as an individualized form of pregnancy treatment – carries a good deal of weight. However, the increased prevalence of medication has led to the introduction of additional regulations on who can distribute abortion pills as well as safeguarding legislation intended to mitigate risks (Romanis and Parsons, 2020; Romanis et al., 2021).

We know that, in the Global South, abortion is often tied to post-abortion care and, historically, wider programmes for family planning built on Malthussian logics of population control (Nandagiri, 2021). While, superficially, this may seem relatively unproblematic, it can impact both the types of abortion services that receive attention and the way that abortion and abortion seekers are treated. Suh (2018) has argued, based on research in Senegal, how the dominance of post-abortion care programmes has orientated abortion politics away from supporting reproductive autonomy to preventing potential mothers from dying and amplifying the risks abortion presents. The bundling of abortion, post-abortion care and family planning, without challenging wider stigmatization of abortion or promoting reproductive justice frameworks that emphasize autonomy, can reinforce the stratification of reproduction services, with abortion positioned as an inherently risky, last resort where family planning has failed.

We know that information governance and provision is a critical part of global abortion politics. The provision of accurate information about pregnancies and about where and how to access abortion care is essential to making abortion access a reality (Drovetta, 2015). Information is increasingly recognized as central to harm reduction (Gill, Cleeve and Lavelanet, 2021). Contrarily, the miscommunication of information about abortion, by accident or intention, has been highlighted as an efficient, and common, way to interrupt access to abortion (Zurek et al., 2015). In some countries, including Australia, New Zealand and the Republic of Ireland, State health services have established and manage safe abortion information hotlines as a way to address impediments to abortion trajectories (Coast et al., 2018).

Pro-choice abortion developments and the interpretation of abortion trails

Taken as a whole, this brief overview is indicative of the general, if consistently contested, orientation towards demedicalizing abortion, pursuing decriminalization and establishing what the WHO addresses as a supportive and enabling environment for safe abortion care (WHO, 2022). This could be interpreted as shaped by the ascendance of rights-based and harm reduction arguments within the abortion context, as well as an increasing awareness, due to the interventions of reproductive justice activists and critical public health scholars, with issues of health inequities. Similarly, it could be viewed as the result of the growth and increased efficacy of health activist movements which aim to disrupt the hegemonic and controlling position of the medical profession in health, as well as address unequal access and underscore issues of rights (Epstein, 2008).

What I want to argue here is that the developments in abortion politics can also be interpreted through a narrative politics lens as reflections of the dominance of specific framings of abortion trails. If we accept that abortion trails, and unsanctioned access to abortion in general, are ontological and that global abortion politics is aware of this – a point which has legitimacy given the circulation of statements regarding the existence of abortion for thousands of years and recognition that abortion is unpreventable – then we must concomitantly appreciate that attitudes to and views on abortion trails have had a formative effect on the present state of abortion politics. Pro-choice abortion politics is, arguably, the product of the construction of abortion trails.

Reassessing the developments within and concerns of abortion politics globally, what becomes clear is not only that abortion trails have had a formative effect but the dominant influence has been an interpretation of abortion trails as risky, threatening and controlled by actors separate from a 'formal', State-sanctioned infrastructure. This manifests, for instance, in the attempts to make the movement of abortion medicines, as well as the medicines themselves, safer or more secure. The emphasis here, while recognizing the possibilities that the shadow infrastructures that have developed to facilitate the use of medications as abortifacients offer in terms of broadening abortion access, is on harm reduction. The implication is that the trails that fall either outside of the parameters of existing regulation or work within gaps between different governed terrains need to be controlled and made subject to surveillance. The expansion of legally permitted telemedicine pathways and associated regulation during Covid-19 in countries such as the UK reflects the trend to interpret abortion trails as risky lifelines used in extremis. Medication abortion had been available, outside and in contravention with legal frameworks, prior to Covid-19. It had also been deemed safe by the World Health Organization. The introduction of telemedicine and self-managed and regulations on these trails was not solely triggered by the possibility of using medication abortion but by the increasingly documented usage – and need to use – a way of accessing abortion that was interpreted as a risk.

A reading of developments in abortion politics as reflective of interpretations of abortion trails as problematic is visible in the rationale for liberalizing abortion access in countries such as the Republic of Ireland, which had one of the most restrictive abortion laws globally until 2018 (De Londras and Enright, 2018). Following the repeal of the Eighth Amendment in 2018, the Irish government publicly stated that it intended to establish and make available abortion services in public hospital and health centres across the country from 1 January 2019. As the then Minister for Health, Simon Harris told a press conference on the day the results of the popular referendum to the repeal the Amendment were announced, 'whereas before we told women to "take the boat", we now tell them to "take our hand"'. Before the referendum, defending his government's commitment to campaigning for repeal, the Republic of Ireland's Taoiseach (Prime Minister) Leo Varadkar presented the need for abortion services in Ireland not only as a public desire – which it was, the majority of people voted in favour of abortion provision – but as necessary for public health need to address the use of unsafe, unsanctioned abortion pills ordered online. In the weeks before the referendum, Varadkar argued that it was 'only a matter of time before a woman dies after taking abortion pills' (McQuinn, 2018).

The Irish case is significant as it shows how developments in expanding abortion were shaped by readings of specific aspects or forms of abortion trails as problematic because they fell outside an abortion-specific regulatory framework. While the import of prohibited medicines as well as the use of abortion pills were illegal in the Republic of Ireland – resulted in seizures of abortion pills by the Health Regulatory Products Authority (for figures see Mishtal et al., 2022) – the existence and use of this technological trail (Calkin and Freeman, 2019) was known for some time prior to either Varadkar's 2018 comments or the support for liberalizing abortion gained significant traction. Moreover, as has been already noted in this book and elsewhere, in the absence of abortion care in Ireland, abortion trails and abortion trail activism had supported access for those living on the island of Ireland for decades prior to 2018. The abortion trails for Irish women were maintained by organizations including the UK-based Liverpool Abortion Support Service, ESCORT, Irish Women's Abortion Support Group, and Abortion Support Network, mobilizations in Ireland such as the Women's Information Network, the Dublin and Cork Abortion Information Campaigns, Need An Abortion Ireland and individual providers offering informal, ad hoc emotional support to abortion travellers.

While abortion trail experiences – and even the names and contact details of activists were frequently shrouded in secrecy, the existence of abortion trails from Ireland to other jurisdictions where abortion was legally available or, more recently, of trails of abortion pills to Ireland was well known. Indeed, writing in 2020, physicians involved in the repeal of the Eighth Amendment published an article in the *British Journal of Obstetrics and Gynaecology* describing their experiences of transitioning from 'working in the shadows' (Mullally et al., 2020). As noted in earlier chapters, there are numerous cultural works referencing abortion travel and the abortion trails from and to the island of Ireland.

The influence of framings of abortion trails as potentially dangerous, legally outside or 'lifelines' offered by pro-choice activists in the narrative and developments of pro-choice abortion politics in Ireland, is also reflected by the lack of attention paid to actors who were not part of activist movements in producing and maintaining abortion trails. As indicated by Mullally et al. (2020) as well as pre-liberalization research on health professionals (Duffy et al., 2018) and reviews of organizations such as Doctors for Choice (Bergen, 2022), health professionals working in Irish public hospitals under the pre-2019 restrictive regime were closely involved in supporting those using abortion trails and sharing information about abortion trails. While referral to abortion services by health professionals above other options (e.g. adoption or continuation of pregnancy) was prohibited under the Regulation of Information (Services outside the State for the Termination of Pregnancies) Act 1995, health care professionals offered emotional and practice support and advice to women travelling for abortion services outside Ireland (Duffy et al., 2018).

The critical point here is that the narrative of Ireland's experiences of liberalization constructs the options available to abortion seekers – abortion trails – as problematic. The objectives of the pro-choice abortion policy and legal reforms were to address the usage of risky abortion trails, controlled by activists outside the parameters of State law, used as 'lifelines' within an otherwise uncaring or unsupportive environment. This narrative was articulated both by political elites, such as the Taoiseach/Prime Minister Leo Varadkar and the then minister for health Simon Harris, and by some pro-choice abortion activists, who used personalized abortion storytelling to amplify the feelings of shame, stigmatization and abandonment felt by those who used abortion trails (Delay and Sundstrom, 2022; Side, 2021).

The pro-choice abortion narrative constituted by these framings of abortion trails amplifies aspects that have been challenged elsewhere. Bobel (2007) for example discusses how a purist vision of activists and activism as taking a separatist form, that is, outside other institutions, does not reflect the diversity of activists. This is further challenged by health social movement writing on 'hybridization' (Roberts et al., 2016) which notes that contemporary mobilizations on health campaigns include actors working within already-regulated institutions (such as the health service). These descriptions tally with the reality of abortion trails connected to the Republic of Ireland which were maintained by health care workers in public hospitals. Moreover, the presentation of abortion trails, which used pills as risky alternatives due to an extreme legal regime, ignored both the evidence supporting the safety of self-managed abortion (including the work of the WHO) and the sophistication of distribution networks. Furthermore, the dominance of a framing of abortion trails as isolating and lonely has been queried by Thomsen (2015) and by abortion trail activists promoting feminist accompaniment and autonomous abortion who argue that these framings reinforce stigmatizing attitudes to abortion and obscure the benefits of using abortion trails for improving the affective experience of abortion (Macón, Solana and Vacarezza, 2021).

Approaching developments in pro-choice abortion politics in Ireland this way suggests that what occurred was not necessarily a demedicalization or shift towards reproductive rights, although the use of rights-arguments was a large component of pro-choice abortion advocacy (Side, 2011; De Londras and Enright, 2018; Carnegie and Roth, 2019). The movement towards liberalization can equally be read as a political manifestation of narrative foreclosures produced by the dominance of specific framings of abortion trails. There are similarities here with this book's opening arguments about how readings of trails orientated political attitudes and interventions. More importantly for abortion politics, the developments in Ireland speak to a constitution of what counts as a 'formal' abortion architecture and how the formalized abortion architecture produced by underscoring abortion trails as external and dangerous orientated the pro-choice abortion movement towards an interpretation of formality as State control. However, based on experiences from countries which have pursued State control, there are important questions to ask regarding the limitations of this approach in terms of progressing the political aspirations of the pro-choice abortion movement. This raises a question mark over whether or why a pro-choice abortion movement pursues or should pursue formalization. The remainder of this chapter will address these points.

What counts as a formal abortion architecture?

Within the narrative politics of abortion, as indicated above, formality is constituted in contexts like the Republic of Ireland as co-ordinated by a health service infrastructure regulated by the State. However, there are questions to be asked here regarding the distinctiveness in real terms of a 'formal' architecture and whether this is constituted by comparison with the actual characteristics of abortion trails or by comparison with the characteristics connected with abortion trails by the narrative framings shaping pro-choice abortion politics. Again, Ireland is a good illustration of this issue as the presentation of the post-2019 service as a formal architecture because it was co-ordinated by Ireland's health services and subject to regulations established by the Irish government through next legislation. However, as noted previously in this chapter, prior to the implementation of this formalized version, abortion trails from, to and within the island of Ireland included components co-ordinated by health services which were, as health care institutions, subject to regulations (Duffy et al., 2018; Bergen, 2022).

Similarly, abortion trails in countries where the majority of abortions are accessed in clandestinity, outside the parameters of a State-managed health service, are supported and include actors who are very much part of a formal health architecture. This is the case in countries in Latin America, including those with stringent anti-abortion regulations, where medications are purchased from pharmacists. Again, the implication that formality is a regulated alternative to a shadow or legally outside abortion trail, is troubled by the fact that abortion trails cut across formal and informal architectures. This 'cutting across' is reflected in both medication abortion trails, which include the participation of health care workers, and in logistical or practical support networks where abortion trails involve accompaniment to formal, State-supported medical centres.

The narrative politics of pro-choice abortion project has, at times, constructed the formal as the anthesis of an informal, 'lifeline' abortion trail. This is certainly the case in the Republic of Ireland. It is also the case in the United States in discussions of abortion care access prior to the 1973 *Roe v Wade* judgement and, more recently, following the Supreme Court's overturning of Roe in the 2022 *Dobbs vs Jackson Women's Health Organization* judgement. The architecture of abortion that operated between these time-points is presented in media coverage and cultural representations, including those of movements such as the Jane Collective, as a more reliable, cohesive infrastructure. Yet, reproductive justice scholars and activists, prior to and following *Dobbs*, highlighted the systemic barriers within this more reliable abortion trail (Luna, 2020) and the disconnected obstacle course facing abortion seekers (Cohen and Joffe, 2020).

What emerges here, based even on these limited examples, is that a formal architecture of abortion is not necessarily either wholly disconnected from or more co-ordinated than abortion trails. That said, it is constituted the framings of abortion trails that are amplified. Applying sociological theory, such as the work of Barad (2007), formality is brought into being through delineation according to normative measures of informality. This position emphasizes the role of discursive separations between manifestations of order and of disorder in the materialization of a formal body.

Additionally, if we follow through sociological contestations of writers such as Sara Ahmed, particularly her work *What's the Use? On the Uses of Use* (Ahmed, 2019), what counts as a formal architecture is defined according to the requirements and desires of colonialist, political elites. In this work, Ahmed contends that the separation between useful and useless objects is based on their legitimacy and value within a colonial capitalist logic as well as their status as owned and managed by colonizers. In relation to the nature of the formal abortion architecture, this foregrounds that the formality of abortion infrastructures in places like Ireland post-2019 is not necessarily constituted by being part of a State health service but by being predominantly or wholly controlled by the State. This is distinct from the pre-2019 or indeed continuing abortion trails which may include actors regulated by the State but are not controlled or directed by the State.

Writing on health social movements, Roberts et al. (2016) articulate the difference between formal and informal in terms of confrontation versus corporatization or collaboration with elite institutions, predominantly State institutions but also the associated biomedical establishment (e.g. health services and clinical medicine).

The delineation is conceptualized through exploring the folding or connectedness of different domains of health and an associated shift not necessarily in organizational membership but in the directing logics and hierarchies of knowledge within formalized domains. Roberts et al. discuss this through considering the changing interests and goals of the National Childbirth Trust (NCT), a UK-based organization established in the 1950s to '[champion] the rights of women to make choices about childbirth' (Roberts et al., 2016: 419) through free-birth or natural-birth. Overtime, the NCT's 'cause' has been reconstituted as addressing the risks associated with lack of access to public health services and expanding the provision of natural or less actively managed (Thornton and Lilford, 1994; Darra, 2009) childbirth within the UK's public health service.

The NCT and orientation of this movement from seeking autonomous childbirth outside the direction of health service managers towards expanding the availability of less actively managed labour within public health services is a useful example of how framings of health care trails constitute an imagining of the formal and, by consequence, the orientation of a rights-based movement towards it. According to Roberts et al.'s reading, the NCT initially amplified the problems of biomedicalized childbirth and sought to establish a cohesive alternative through collaborations between lay activists and medical professionals. From the 2000s on, however, the dominant risks/problems underscored included the absence of State-controlled pathways to natural childbirth and need to get advice on health care needs, for example breastfeeding, from sources outside UK health services. The narrative of the NCT's cause altered from addressing restrictions to making different childbirth choices and infant care practices safer through the State actively taking control of these health services.

Limitations of a formal architecture

Although the introduction of a more liberal abortion care regime in the Republic of Ireland undoubtedly expanded the ability of women living in Ireland to access abortion and removed the burden of abortion travel for the majority of abortion seekers, the formalized architecture of abortion care is neither as equitable nor as responsive to the needs of marginalized groups as the abortion trail. Formalization has, research undertaken since the introduction of services demonstrates, not addressed the additional impediments facing migrants (Chakravarty et al., 2023), marginalized communities or people seeking later abortions (Grimes et al., 2023). The distribution of services across Ireland is not even, resulting in geographic inequality in terms of care (Duffy, Freeman and Rodriguez, 2023).

Furthermore, similar to diversity management approaches criticized by Anthias (2013), the formal architecture of abortion care is orientated towards supporting a 'tolerable' spectrum of abortion care subjectivities. This is reflected in the support, or rather the limited support, available for those attempting to access abortion at a later gestation for maternal health reasons or the exclusion of foetal anomalies which would not definitively lead to the death of the foetus in utero or twenty-eight days post-partum (Grimes et al., 2023). The upshot of these conditionalities within the formal abortion care infrastructure was the increase in abortion travel by women living in Ireland seeking abortion for foetal anomaly or maternal health reasons or later abortion (Miremberg et al., 2023; Duffy, Freeman and Rodriguez, 2023; O'Shea, 2023). The newly-introduced formal architecture of abortion, adapting Side's (2021) contentions on how abortion laws introduce borders between permissible and impermissible abortion, arguably 'rebordered' abortion around schemas of acceptability. This reflects a form of reproductive governance (Morgan and Roberts, 2012), instituting a stratified framework of reproductive autonomy (Kimport, Weitz and Freedman, 2016) according to perspectives on permissible abortion as compared with unacceptable or transgressive abortion (Nandagiri and Pizzarossa, 2023).

Ireland is not alone in demonstrating the limitations of a 'formal' architecture. Uneven access to abortion was also visible in the extended formal abortion care system in Colombia following 2006. Prior to a 2006 judgement by the Corte Constitucional, abortion was illegal in

Colombia in almost all circumstances, with high rates of clandestine abortions, using abortion trails common (Stifani et al., 2018). While the Corte's judgement expanded the ability of care providers, including providers in hospitals covered by public health insurance, to support abortion seekers through emphasizing human rights interpretations of health and well-being, the increasingly formal infrastructure of care did not comprehensively challenge the stigmatizing attitudes towards abortion or lack of understanding of abortion rights that activists highlighted as it resulted in abortion seekers relying on clandestine, shadow infrastructures. Pro-abortion groups such as La Mesa Por La Vida, Orientamé and Las Parceras, following the 2006 judgement continued to work to both support abortion seekers and push against the barriers they were able to report through individual applications to the Constitutional Court (under the *tutela* system). In 2021, their actions, brought together under a collective action of hundreds of activists and pro-choice abortion advocates and allies (the *Causa Justa*), resulted in the decriminalization of abortion up to twenty-four-weeks' gestation.

Yet, as interviewees for the research underpinning this book, in research undertaken prior decriminalization, emphasized, the formal abortion care system in Colombia after 2006 remained heavily weighted against those in isolated areas, living in poverty or accessing abortion in hospitals. All of these persistent problems were outlined by a pro-choice advocate at a health care centre in Bogotá who described the reality of accessing sexual and reproductive health care in Colombia in the following way:

> Yo siento que la salud sexual y reproductiva en Colombia todavía sigue siendo el privilegio de muy pocas mujeres en el país [...] Entonces esto se debe a muchas barreras o factores que impiden que la gente acceda libremente a la prestación de los servicios de salud. Primero, una gran barrera es el acceso en general al sistema y a los servicios de salud, teniendo en cuenta como la gran cantidad de desempleo, los índices de desempleo tan altos generan que esto ya se constituya en una primera barrera de acceso, porque empiezan a formar parte del sistema del régimen subsidiado de salud que, sin estimgatizar y sin generar como

polarización frente a esto le da un cierto componente de límite al acceso. [. . .] Las condiciones socio económicas del país que impiden que la gente esté afiliada al sistema de seguridad social ensalud y de ahí las barreras frente a los derechos sexuales y reproductivos. Accesibilidad por ubicación geográfica, accesibilidad por falta de información. Las personas en el país todavía no son coscientes o tal vez no saben que la materialización de los derechos sexuales y reproductivos, en la garantía de la situación sexual y reproductiva, es muy importante.

I feel that sexual and reproductive health care in Colombia is still the privilege of a very small number of women in the country [. . .] So, this is due to many barriers or factors that prevent people from freely accessing health services provided. First, a big barrier is access in general to the health system and services, taking into account the large number of unemployed people, the very high rates of unemployment mean that this already constitutes a first barrier, because they rely on a subsidized health system which, without stigmatising or polarizing, gives a certain degree of limiting access. [. . .] The socio-economic circumstances in the country that prevent people from being affiliated with a health social security system and hence the barriers to sexual and reproductive rights. Accessibility due to geographic location, accessibility due to lack of information. People in the country are still unaware or perhaps unaware that the materialization of sexual and reproductive rights, in guaranteeing sexual and reproductive rights, is very important.
   (Pro-choice advocate, Bogotá, TN107; my translation)

The formalization of abortion care was also unaccompanied by efforts to compel regional health care commissioners to establish and sustain provision through public hospitals. This resulted in instances of conservative, religiously managed, hospitals claiming 'institutional conscience objection' and refusing to provide abortion services. Furthermore, Catholic universities refused to permit those undertaking medical degrees at their institutions to learn how to perform abortion care. This created, as the interviewee above noted, a situation, within subsidized or public health settings in particular, where '*la prestación de los servicios quizás está permeada por la incapacidad del talento humano*' (translation: the provision of services is permeated by a lack of human talent/personnel; interviewee TN107).

What links both the formal infrastructures of care which expanded in Ireland and Colombia following legal change is the absence of attempts to disrupt the inequalities and barriers to care. What Colombia and Ireland indicate is that the process of constructing a formal abortion care infrastructure supported by the State and led by medical institutions may neither address nor rectify pronounced forms of disadvantage experienced by some abortion seekers. It is notable in both these instances that the process of drawing abortion out of the shadows did not work in tandem with a critical assessment of the political economies of health within either country. This is despite the fact that much of the work of abortion trail activism is dedicated towards supporting those at a financial disadvantage or who do not have local access to abortion services. Equally interesting is the absence of a concerted, State-supported attempt to address attitudes to abortion within the health profession. In Ireland, values clarification was initiated by health providers who had been involved for the campaign for the repeal of the Eighth Amendment and largely delivered on a voluntary basis by committed providers supported by the World Health Organization (Bergen, 2022; Mishtal et al., 2022). In Colombia, abortion training is provided by private clinics, such as Profamilia and Orientamé, rather than through State-financed medical training programmes.

Although access to abortion certainly expanded in both jurisdictions following legal changes, the extent to which the discourse of abortion as a private, medicalized, treatment that was acceptable under limited circumstances but ultimately morally dubious was challenged by establishing a formal architecture of abortion care or expanding the ability of the existing architecture to provide abortion care is questionable. Applying Ahmed (2019), this reflects a non-performative approach rather than the adoption of a phenomenological attitude. The interest of the State is not reproductive autonomy or meaningfully addressing potential impediments to abortion access through transformative change. Rather it is in managing, and making manageable and governable, a means of accessing abortion that exists and operates independently of the State. This competing interest was made explicit during the campaigns in advance of legal change in Ireland where a significant emphasis was placed on the need to regulate for abortion to eradicate a dangerous backstreet of self-managed abortion using illegally imported medicines.

Conclusion: Why pursue formalization?

The discussion above points to a clear tension within the orientation of pro-choice abortion politics towards establishing or expanding a State-controlled, formal abortion architecture. Not only does it require the amplification of framings of abortion trails as risky and only used as 'lifelines' where a legal framework either does not exist or works against abortion, it also has limitations in terms of enabling equitable abortion access. Why seek control of abortion trails by the State? It would be straightforward, and legitimate, at this point to present the narrative constitution of partially State-controlled abortion trail as 'informal' and foreclosure of abortion trails as undesirable by an orientation towards formalization as illustrative of dominance of a liberal, choice-based interpretation of reproductive rights. This, as Thomsen (2015) notes, is a central argument of reproductive justice narratives.

As a conclusion to this and the preceding chapters' discussion about how foregrounding abortion trails can assist analyse and expand our understanding of the pro-choice abortion project, I wish to trouble this interpretation of why pro-choice movements pursue collaboration with the State or formalization. Again, narrative politics are relevant here as my aim is to highlight the potential for reading the constitution of pro-choice abortion politics towards State-sanctioned abortion architectures or State-guaranteed rights not as reflective of the emphasis on the dangers of abortion trails but of the emphasis on the advanced and progressive practices circulating within the shadows. In short, I want to propose an alternative reading of why a pro-choice project may pursue, or be constituted as pursuing, the absorption and State control of abortion trails. My contention here is based on literature on health activism which presents part of the 'cause' (O'Donovan, Moreira and Howlett, 2013) of health social movements as challenging the exclusion of practices and knowledges generated by those involved in practices of improving embodied experiences or care needs from legitimate sites or discourses of health care. Formalization can be framed as the result of the amplification of health trails as external, alternative, or lifelines and the presentation of these qualities as risky or dangerous. However, it can equally be interpreted as constituted by the successful breakthrough of lay activists involved in what Diedrich (2013) discusses as 'que(er)ying care' and the Care Collective (2020), a group of UK scholars writing on the politics of care and interdependency, present as 'promiscuous care' (i.e. care provided by strangers in informal ways) into a field of social and political relations underpinned by biomedical hegemony.

It is possible to suggest that an argument for formalization is to encourage medical elites and State-controlled institutions learn form and take advantage of the expertise and skills developed within abortion trails (envisaged as a shadow infrastructure). This argument is found within writing on health social movements strategies which highlights that the constitution and orientation of advocacy groups towards collaboration is not illustrative of supplanting resistant activism with State control (Roberts et al., 2016). Rather it was part of a strategy of emphasizing the legitimacy of lay expertise and challenging the framing of non-State health actors as ill-informed and uncoordinated. The orientation towards formalization can be interpreted as part of a politics of potentialities (Ganchoff, 2004) for generating new forms of health care which meaningfully collaborated and learned from embodied knowledge.

However, in the case of Ireland, what became almost immediately apparent was that the process of formalizing abortion trails would not involve integrating the attentiveness to feminist care ethics or intent to generate a health care landscape which recognized and supported all reproductive health journeys. More worryingly for abortion trail activists committed to autonomous abortion care, infrastructures outside of State health settings or which allowed self-management without connecting with clinicians were not permitted under the formalized abortion architecture. The aspiration that formalization would actively bring together lay expertise and State-controlled medical institutions in generative ways, in Roberts et al. (2016), that folding the confrontational and the corporate with help the abortion trail activists strengthen their position and the abortion trail as a site of developing knowledge that was viewed as a legitimate participate within health policy spaces (Ganchoff, 2004) did not transpire. Indeed, the new law on abortion – the Health [Regulation of Termination of Pregnancy Services] Act 2019 – explicitly legislated against and introduced criminal sanctions directly targeted at a shadow infrastructure.

The key point to take away from this experience is not that the orientation towards a State-controlled abortion architecture cannot be interpreted as an effect of framing abortion trails as a shadow infrastructure. Rather it is that a continued pursuit of this goal ignores the tendency of State institutions to limit the capacity of trails to continue to generate new ways of thinking or meaningfully alter discourse once they assumed control of trails.

Conclusion

The thing about being a pro-choice activist is that, perhaps unsurprisingly, people want to talk to me about abortion. A lot. People will tell me their own abortion stories or ones they've heard. I've had friends of friends tell me stories of how they've travelled on their own with barely enough money to have an abortion in an English clinic. [. . .]

Sometimes though, someone will come to me in crisis and ask for advice on how to arrange their abortion because they don't know how to navigate such things. How would they? It's not something anyone plans for. There is no organization out there you can ring and say, 'Hey, I'm in Ireland. I'm in a crisis pregnancy situation, please make the requisite arrangements for me. You can start with getting me the days off work and booking my flights'.

Stephanie Lord, *The Logistics of Arranging Abortions*

They did not wait for the law to change, but rather took the necessary initiatives . . .

Sandra Jeppesen and Holly Nazar, *Genders and Sexualities in Anarchist Movements*

Her ma said, 'Here, c'mere, c'mere, c'mere
Look listen, understand there's no money for a trip on the ringer,
that's only for those that can.'

Emmet Kirwan, *Heartbreak*

[La Red Compañera, Red Latinamericana y Caribeña de Acompañantes de aborto] *es una apuesta colectiva, amorosa, rebelde y llena de resistencia feminista, para acompañar abortos en diversas latitudes, para resignificarlos y poner en el centro a quienes abortan*

[La Red Compañera, Red Latinamericana y Caribeña de Acompañantes de aborto] is a commitment to collective, loving, rebellious and fully

feminist resistance to accompany abortion in various places, to give new meaning to them, and to put those who abort at the centre
Laura Rosso (author's translation in italics)

For some time now, I have been thinking about getting an abortion. Not, strictly speaking, from a personal perspective. I have never sought an abortion (although it may be possible that, in my remaining time of being of gestational age, I may need to do so). I am from the Global North, from a country (the Republic of Ireland) where a constitutional amendment that recognized the right to life of the unborn was inserted following a popular referendum before I was born. While this provision – the Eighth Amendment – did not originally contain the word abortion, it created a medico-legal environment where there was a presumption towards continuation of a pregnancy to birth and acted as a de facto anti-abortion law for over thirty years (De Londras and Enright, 2018; Enright and Duffy, 2022; Fitzsimons, 2021). I have also researched the impact of this anti-abortion law, and its repeal in 2018, on the perceptions of health care professionals and health services in Ireland (Duffy et al., 2018; Mishtal et al., 2022; Duffy, Freeman and Rodriguez, 2023).

I have lived in Liverpool, a key destination for abortion travel from Ireland or, to use the poet Emmet Kirwan's words 'took a trip on the ringer'. I have given birth, thankfully without any substantial difficulties, three times at Liverpool Women's Hospital, a hospital which, as well as being one of the largest dedicated centres for obstetrics and gynaecology care in the north-west of England, was given a memorial by the Irish campaigning and support group Termination for Medical Reasons for the support given by bereavement support teams to Irish patients who could not legally access care 'at home'. The actor, Brian F. O'Byrne, in his acceptance speech for a 2018 British Academy of Film and Television Award (BAFTA) also thanked 'the Women's' (to give the hospital its local moniker), 'for looking after my fellow Irish citizens, who come there in distress, daily. Thank you, Britain, for looking after our women in their time of need' (Gorman, 2018). As I noted within this book, Liverpool occupies a key position in Irish histories of both migration and abortion. From the late 1970s onwards, feminist activists in and beyond Liverpool have openly mobilized to support women travelling from Ireland seeking abortion through organizations such as the Liverpool Abortion Support Service, ESCORT and the Abortion Support Network (Duffy, 2020; Fletcher, 2016). Contrary to Stephanie Lord's comments that there was 'no organisation that [you] can ring' to support the logistics of abortion access for women living in Ireland, there were a number of groups, in Ireland and abroad, who positioned themselves as providing exactly this form of support.

Moreover, for most of my adult life, I have lived in Britain, in England, where over 200,000 women from Ireland have accessed abortions since the implementation of the Abortion Act 1967. Abortion statistics also indicate that England is an abortion travel destination for people living in other European countries, in liberal and illiberal regimes (Garnsey et al., 2021; Gerdts et al., 2016). Although the Abortion Act 1967 was never extended to Northern Ireland (Pierson and Bloomer, 2017), and despite the geographic disparities in abortion access in Britain (Lohr et al., 2022), realities which challenge a framing of the UK as an 'abortion-providing' country, I have found it extremely interesting how far removed many English people distance themselves from the idea of abortion as restricted or contingent. This is despite the fact that the Abortion Act is a 'grounds-based' legislation which permits abortion under specific circumstances, with confirmation from and under supervision of two doctors. The requirements of the legislation, and their stringent implementation, have resulted in criminal charges being brought against those who have self-managed abortion outside the permissible boundaries of the law. Furthermore, since its introduction, both the Abortion Act 1967 and abortion services have been targeted by anti-choice campaigners. Challenges have taken the form of direct protests outside clinics (Lowe and Page, 2022) as well as restrictions on points of access and legislative challenges on gestational limits (Sheldon et al., 2022).

I have therefore reflected from three positions: one where I am keenly aware of the capacity of the State to restrict abortion; one where I am aware of the persistent contingencies and precarity of abortion access within countries where abortion access is assumed as immutable or where the State has been pursued to guarantee abortion access; and one where I am conscious that groups and individuals often, in direct contravention with the law (Jeppesen and Nazar, 2012), facilitate abortion care both in circumstances where abortion is not provided for by health services or reproductive law and policy or where the State, medical institutions and social attitudes actively work in opposition to abortion access. These groups and individuals act in a range of ways and contexts and take a variety of organizational forms. Yet despite their essential status for some abortion seekers and long history, they are frequently treated descriptively or become subject to efforts to categorize their work and interests (i.e. as practical support, as abortion pill networks or as abortion funds). Research tends to use the labels that activists and organizations use. This is obviously important in terms of reflecting how collectives define themselves but it can create challenges for a broader discussion about their shared identity as a form of political praxis.

The issue here is how to move from the descriptive to the discursive and the analytic – how to explore the resonant political logics and interests of groups while still recognizing their inherent diversity. This book proceeded from this position, adopting a term that speaks to both nebulousness and distinguishable characteristics – abortion trail activism. It aimed to use this term to consider the shared intentions of the diverse mobilizations as illustrative of a distinct political intervention. It further presented abortion trail activism as analytically useful to draw attention to the narrative politics of pro-choice abortion activism, what shapes the orientation of the pro-choice abortion project, what divergences within this project abortion trail activism can underscore as well as the limitations of some ways the pro-choice abortion project has been pursued (specifically the control of abortion trails by the State).

Why abortion trail activism?

Part of the attraction of abortion trail activism above practical support network, abortion travel, medical tourism, abortion mobilities or autonomous health organization is the ambivalence of the term trail. From a sociological perspective, a trail is an assemblage of material and non-material objects, practices and things. Moor writes about trails as having a 'soul', as an interlocutor between use and memory. Trails have also been documented, analysed and translated in ways that carry and convey vastly different inflections. Bachelard presents trails as *les chemins du désir* – lines of desire – connecting space, use and want. This conveys a wishful and hopeful sensation. Yet trails can also be adequately translated as *panya* ('rat routes'), 'backstreets' or 'county lines', none of which automatically carry the same aspirational and happier hues as desire lines. That said, depending on ones' social, economic, embodied and classed position, these apparently riskier trails can represent or facilitate a more autonomous life where conduct is less subject to State surveillance and control.

Trails also hold an attraction because of their relationship with time and temporality. Trails have a history and a memory (Luckert, 2012), and while we may romanticize trailblazers or those who forge trails, we are keenly aware that trails are constructed through collective enterprise. The persistence of trails cannot be attributed to one individual, working alone. There is also a sense that some trails have no fixed beginning or chronology, and certainly not one that could be traced definitively. Trails become visible as we encounter them but also can recede from view and, without continued use or preservation, disappear entirely. Simultaneously, trails can be made governable through intervention. They can precede, direct and be claimed by formal borders. Trails can become subject to protect and regulate orders if recognized as having cultural or economic value.

Trails, arguably, have an (un)timeliness. Trails are used when needed – either because the time requires a trail or our actions or presence needs to be made more timely. They thus have a timeliness. But they also enable us to preserve or dispense with time and are equally untimely. We can gain haste or allow ourselves to be unhastened by entering into or using a trail. The existence of a trail can permit, by default, the abdication of responsibility or will to become more timely or adapt to the times better.

It is the effervescent character of trail that makes it a useful device for discussing the multiple forms of activism and varying movements that, in this volume, I have connected together under the heading 'abortion trail activism'. Just as the definition of trail brings together use and desire, history and immediacy, as well as formal and subversive, abortion trail activism contains multiple meanings. There is no single, pure abortion trail.

Ultimately, I have aimed to present abortion trail activism as a distinguishable form of abortion activism, underpinned by identifiable commitments and ideologies. Having established these commitments and ideologies, I then sought to interrogate the position of abortion trail activism within the terrain of pro-choice mobilizing. I was, and remain, particularly interested in what foregrounding abortion trail activism as an analytic focal point contributes to unpacking the pro-choice abortion narrative and the orientation the pro-choice project towards a formal, State-sanctioned and medicalized infrastructure of abortion care.

To conclude the discussions within this volume, I want to underscore the key arguments that can be gleaned from scrutinizing abortion trail activism, as I have attempted to do. I also want to identify some orientations for ongoing conversations both of abortion trail activism and the global pro-choice project.

Understanding abortion trail activism

This book was principally dedicated to enriching understandings of abortion trail activism. With regard to this objective, the analysis presented in the preceding chapters brings us to the following conclusions:

1. Abortion trail activism is a fundamentally practical political project dedicated at addressing the accessibility of abortion. As such it combines a range of tactics and engagements directed at addressing barriers and facilitators to abortion. These respond to and are shaped by human and non-human factors, ranging from perceptions about abortion to the physical location of clinics or pharmacies.
2. Abortion trails and abortion trail activism are neither synonymous nor mutually exclusive. There are well-worn paths to abortion that exist independently of abortion trail activism; at the same time, there are examples of collective actions by abortion trail activists establishing a trail.
3. Abortion trail activism is inspired by a feminist ethic of care. Feminist ethics approaches care as ontological, relational, affective and is shaped by and produces particular subjectivities, knowledges, beliefs and power relations. From this understanding, feminist ethics of care advocates and pursues non-normative, resistant and more equitable caring practices, experiences and relationships.
4. Consistent with its feminist ethic, abortion trail activism emphasizes the ontological character of abortion and critiques normative readings of abortion. Instead it focuses on addressing the ways care can reinforce systems of power within discourses of care.
5. Abortion trail activism is a prefigurative politics. The actions abortion trail activists engage in are experiments in constructing a transformative imagining of abortion care in the present.

The analytic value of abortion trail activism

As well as presenting abortion trail activism as a mechanism for distinguishing and connecting a specific political praxis, the book aimed to underscore the analytic usefulness of foregrounding abortion trails activism when thinking about the orientation of the pro-choice abortion project. This was the focus of Chapters 4 and 5, in which I argued that abortion trails can illuminate the narrative politics and political contestations within the pro-choice abortion project. Specifically, thinking through trails can show how the framings of abortion trails have constitutive effects on what a formal architecture of abortion care looks like and on the orientation of pro-choice abortion mobilizations.

This part of the book presents a different understanding of what has shaped pro-choice abortion politics than that suggested by either reproductive justice or reproductive rights scholars, both of whom, by way of description (reproductive rights) or critique (reproductive justice), present pro-choice abortion politics as influenced by a foregrounding of individualized rights. Through using abortion trails as an analytic starting point, this section of the book proposed that the pro-choice abortion project was shaped by the framing of abortion trails. This explains why the pro-choice abortion project can pursue State-sanctioning of abortion architectures while at the same time knowing that the State is a problematic actor. In this instance, collaboration with or the absorption of abortion trails is seen as strategically desirable in order to centre and promote the expertise generated in abortion trails within the State-run, biomedical systems of abortion health care.

Abortion trail activism and the pro-choice project

A central theme within this book has been what directly analysing abortion trail activism can reveal about the pro-choice project. Within the preceding chapters, I outlined how abortion trail activism drew attention to the amplification within pro-choice narratives of the danger and precarity of abortion trails without recognizing with regard to the equality problematic realities of abortion care access in State-controlled abortion systems. Through the examples of the Republic of Ireland after 2019 and Colombia between 2006 and 2022, I identified how comparison of the formalized abortion care infrastructures with the abortion trail activism/shadow infrastructure highlighted the exclusions of formalization and, by association, the pro-choice project.

Specifically, I argued that a pro-choice abortion project that sought State control of abortion provision without pursuing the commitments of abortion trail activism – to ensure abortion care's accessibility, to establish an infrastructure of abortion care underpinned by feminist ethics and to operate prefiguratively – would reinforce the acute problems experienced by those most disadvantaged by anti-abortion law and policy. This includes materially disadvantaged communities – in terms of economic deprivation and absence of transport links or health services – as well as migrants, ethnic minorities and those seeking abortions at a later stage or for reasons deemed less morally acceptable.

Looking at examples when the pro-choice abortion project has pursued establishing a formal, State-controlled architecture also indicates what sutured into abortion care when States assume control of providing abortion completely. These included contingencies of access as well as an additional political economy of abortion where accessibility was facilitated or limited through the organization of health services. Additional regulations, on who could support abortion, what support should look like and where abortion support can happen, are woven into the architecture of abortion care as the State replaces abortion trail activists. Within a context where health care is predominantly provided by medics and clinicians, this can result in a medicalization of abortion care, an outcome that can undermine reproductive autonomy.

By considering the exclusions within a formalized pro-choice abortion care architecture, this book offers an indication as to what the future orientation of the pro-abortion care project should be. This is of pronounced importance at the present moment when the terrain of gender health care politics in some, previously liberal, abortion care regimes (particularly the United States and England and Wales) is shifting towards legal and political positions that run counter to the aspirations of abortion trail activists.

However, it is perhaps less helpful to dictate what the global pro-choice project should prioritize based on what some States have excluded. A more productive approach is to look to abortion trail activism as a framework of what abortion care can and should look like. This carries the additional benefits of valuing abortion care activism as fully as it deserves as well as recognizing that abortion trails are continuously remade regardless of the existence of a formal abortion pathway.

So, what can abortion trail activism teach us about how to proceed? In the first instance, abortion trail activism demonstrates the importance of considering care critically – what is the type of abortion care we would like to see? If it respects reproductive autonomy, wants to transform the affective experience of having an abortion and is committed to disrupting the barriers that abortion seekers can, and regularly do, encounter, then a model of abortion care underpinned by the commitments of abortion trail activism is ultimately more desirable. Because, above all, surely the abortion care we desire most is one that is care-full, accessible and resistant to the imposition of conditions. As *acompañante* activists and allies like Laura Rosso, cited at this chapter's opening, assert – we desire abortions free from constraints and abortions filled with love.

Bibliography

Ackerman, Edwin. '"What Part of Illegal Don't You Understand?":
  Bureaucracy and Civil Society in the Shaping of Illegality'. *Ethnic and
  Racial Studies* 37, no. 2 (2014): 181–203.
Ahmed, Sara. *On Being Included: Racism and Diversity in Institutional Life*.
  London: Duke University Press, 2012.
Ahmed, Sara. *The Promise of Happiness*. London: Duke University Press, 2020.
Ahmed, Sara. *What's the Use?: On the Uses of Use*. London: Duke University
  Press, 2019.
Aiken, Abigail R. A., Jennifer E. Starling, Rebecca Gomperts, James G. Scott,
  and Catherine E. Aiken. 'Demand for Self-Managed Online Telemedicine
  Abortion in Eight European Countries during the COVID-19 Pandemic:
  A Regression Discontinuity Analysis'. *BMJ Sexual & Reproductive Health*
  47, no. 4 (2021): 238–45.
Akinbola, Bimbola. '# AfricanAunties: Performing Diasporic Digital
  Disbelongings on TikTok'. *Text and Performance Quarterly* 42, no. 3
  (2022): 284–97.
Alam, Ashraful and Donna Houston. 'Rethinking Care as Alternate
  Infrastructure'. *Cities* 100 (2020): 102662.
Albrecht, Gary L., Katherine D. Seelman, and Michael Bury. London:
  Handbook of Disability Studies. Sage, 2001.
Anthias, Floya. 'Moving beyond the Janus Face of Integration and Diversity
  Discourses: Towards an Intersectional Framing'. *The Sociological Review*
  61, no. 2 (2013): 323–43.
Anzaldúa, Gloria. 'To Live in the Borderlands'. In *The Multicultural Southwest:
  A Reader*, edited by A. Gabriel Mélendez, M. Jane Young, Patricia Moore,
  and Patrick Pynes, 139–40. Tucson: University of Arizona Press, 1987.
Ashe, Muesiri O. and Vivian B. Ojong. 'Border Management and Gender
  Issues in Sub-Saharan Africa's Cross-Border Trade under COVID-19'.
  African Journal of Gender, Society & Development 11, no. 1 (2022): 33–53.
Assifi, Anisa R., Melissa Kang, Elizabeth A. Sullivan, and Angela J. Dawson.
  'Abortion Care Pathways and Service Provision for Adolescents in High-

Income Countries: A Qualitative Synthesis of the Evidence'. *PLoS One* 15, no. 11 (2020): e0242015.
Assis, Mariana Prandini. 'Liberating Abortion Pills in Legally Restricted Settings 1: Activism as Public Criminology'. In *Routledge Handbook of Public Criminologies*, edited by Kathryn Henne and Rita Shah, 120–30. New York: Routledge, 2020.
Assis, Mariana Prandini and Joanna N. Erdman. 'Abortion Rights beyond the Medico-Legal Paradigm'. *Global Public Health* 17, no. 10 (2022): 2235–50.
Bachelard, Gaston. *The Poetics of Space*. New York :Penguin, 2014.
Ballakrishnen, Swethaa S. 'Anti/Aunty as Critical Method: From Gendered Resistance to Soft Grace'. *South Asia: Journal of South Asian Studies* 46, no. 1 (2023): 135–51.
Barad, Karen. *Meeting the Universe Halfway: Quantum Physics and the Entanglement of Matter and Meaning* . London : Duke University Press, 2007.
Barad, Karen. 'Posthumanist Performativity: Toward an Understanding of How Matter Comes to Matter'. *Signs: Journal of Women in Culture and Society* 28, no. 3 (2003): 801–31.
Barry, Ursula. 'Abortion in the Republic of Ireland'. *Feminist Review* 29, no. 1 (1988): 57–63.
Berer, Marge. 'Abortion Law and Policy around the World: In Search of Decriminalization'. *Health and Human Rights* 19, no. 1 (2017): 13.
Bergen, Sadie. '"The Kind of Doctor Who Doesn't Believe Doctor Knows Best": Doctors for Choice and the Medical Voice in Irish Abortion Politics, 2002–2018'. *Social Science & Medicine* 297 (2022): 114817.
Berlant, Lauren. 'Cruel Optimism: On Marx, Loss and the Senses'. *New Formations* 63 (2007): 33.
Berlant, Lauren. *Cruel Optimism*. London: Duke University Press, 2020.
Berro Pizzarossa, Lucía and Rishita Nandagiri. 'Self-Managed Abortion: A Constellation of Actors, a Cacophony of Laws?'. *Sexual and Reproductive Health Matters* 29, no. 1 (2021): 23–30.
Bhardwaj, Maya. 'Bad Brown Aunties, Fagony Aunts and Resistance Aunties: Centring Queer Desi Aunties in Diasporic Social Movement and Justice Work'. *South Asia: Journal of South Asian Studies* 46, no. 1 (2023): 113–34.
Bloomer, Fiona and Emma Campbell, eds. *Decriminalizing Abortion in Northern Ireland: Allies and Abortion Provision*. London, New York: Bloomsbury Publishing, 2022.

Bloomer, Fiona and Kellie O'Dowd. 'Restricted Access to Abortion in the Republic of Ireland and Northern Ireland: Exploring Abortion Tourism and Barriers to Legal Reform'. *Culture, Health & Sexuality* 16, no. 4 (2014): 366–80.

Bloomer, Fiona, Claire Pierson, and Sylvia Claudio Estrada. *Reimagining Global Abortion Politics*. Bristol: Policy Press, 2018.

Boateng, Linda, Mary Nicolaou, Henriëtte Dijkshoorn, Karien Stronks, and Charles Agyemang. 'An Exploration of the Enablers and Barriers in Access to the Dutch Healthcare System among Ghanaians in Amsterdam'. *BMC Health Services Research* 12 (2012): 1–11.

Bobel, Chris. '"I'm Not an Activist, Though I've Done a Lot of It": Doing Activism, being Activist and the "Perfect Standard" in a Contemporary Movement'. *Social Movement Studies* 6, no. 2 (2007): 147–59.

Boggs, Carl. 'Marxism, Prefigurative Communism, and the Problem of Workers' Control'. *Radical America* 11, no. 6 (1977): 99–122.

Bowlby, Sophie. 'Recognising the Time—Space Dimensions of Care: Caringscapes and Carescapes'. *Environment and Planning A* 44, no. 9 (2012): 2101–18.

Braine, Naomi and Marissa Velarde. 'Self-Managed Abortion: Strategies for Support by a Global Feminist Movement'. *Women's Reproductive Health* 9, no. 3 (2022): 183–202.

Braun, Virginia and Victoria Clarke. 'One Size Fits All? What Counts as Quality Practice in (Reflexive) Thematic Analysis?'. *Qualitative Research in Psychology* 18, no. 3 (2021): 328–52.

Braun, Virginia and Victoria Clarke. 'Reflecting on Reflexive Thematic Analysis'. *Qualitative Research in Sport, Exercise and Health* 11, no. 4 (2019): 589–97.

Braun, Virginia and Victoria Clarke. 'Using Thematic Analysis in Psychology'. *Qualitative Research in Psychology* 3, no. 2 (2006): 77–101.

Brown, Phil and Stephen Zavestoski. 'Social Movements in Health: An Introduction'. *Sociology of Health & Illness* 26, no. 6 (2004): 679–94.

Burton, Julia. 'Prácticas feministas en torno al derecho al aborto en Argentina: Aproximaciones a las acciones colectivas de Socorristas en Red'. *Revista Punto Género* 7 (2017): 91–111.

Calkin, Sydney. 'Towards a Political Geography of Abortion'. *Political Geography* 69 (2019): 22–9.

Calkin, Sydney. *Abortion Pills Go Global: Reproductive Freedom Across Borders*. Vol. 7. Oakland, CA: University of California Press, 2023.

Calkin, Sydney and Cordelia Freeman. 'Trails and Technology: Social and Cultural Geographies of Abortion Access'. *Social & Cultural Geography* 20, no. 9 (2019): 1325–32.

Calkin, Sydney, Cordelia Freeman, and Francesca Moore. 'The Geography of Abortion: Discourse, Spatiality and Mobility'. *Progress in Human Geography* 46, no. 6 (2022): 1413–30.

Campbell, E., N. Connor, S. Heaney, and F. Bloomer. 'Training Abortion Doulas in Northern Ireland: Lessons from a COVID-19 Context'. *BMJ Sexual & Reproductive Health* 47, no. 4 (2021): np.

Carel, Havi and Ian James Kidd. 'Epistemic Injustice in Healthcare: A Philosophical Analysis'. *Medicine, Health Care and Philosophy* 17 (2014): 529–40.

Carnegie, Anna and Rachel Roth. 'From the Grassroots to the Oireachtas: Abortion Law Reform in the Republic of Ireland'. *Health and Human Rights* 21, no. 2 (2019): 109.

Carse, Ashley, and David Kneas. 'Unbuilt and Unfinished: The Temporalities of Infrastructure'. *Environment and Society* 10, no. 1 (2019): 9–28.

Center for Reproductive Rights. *World's Abortion Laws Map*. Center for Reproductive Rights, 2021. https://reproductiverights.org/maps/worlds-abortion-laws/ (accessed 30 January 2024).

Chakravarty, Dyuti, Joanna Mishtal, Lorraine Grimes, Karli Reeves, Bianca Stifani, Deirdre Duffy, Mark Murphy, et al. 'Restrictive Points of Entry into Abortion Care in Ireland: A Qualitative Study of Expectations and Experiences with the Service'. *Sexual and Reproductive Health Matters* 31, no. 1 (2023): 2215567.

Chatzidakis, Andreas, Jamie Hakim, Jo Litter, and Catherine Rottenberg. *The Care Manifesto: The Politics of Interdependence*. London: Verso Books, 2020.

Chełstowska, Agata and Agata Ignaciuk. 'Criminalization, Medicalization, and Stigmatization: Genealogies of Abortion Activism in Poland'. *Signs: Journal of Women in Culture and Society* 48, no. 2 (2023): 423–53.

Chiweshe, Malvern, and Catriona Macleod. 'Cultural De-colonization Versus Liberal Approaches to Abortion in Africa: The Politics of Representation and Voice'. *African Journal of Reproductive Health* 22, no. 2 (2018): 49–59.

Chuma, Jane and Vincent Okungu. 'Viewing the Kenyan Health System through an Equity Lens: Implications for Universal Coverage'. *International Journal for Equity in Health* 10 (2011): 1–14.

Cloatre, Emilie and Máiréad Enright. '"On the Perimeter of the Lawful": Enduring Illegality in the Irish Family Planning Movement, 1972–1985'. *Journal of Law and Society* 44, no. 4 (2017): 471–500.

Coast, Ernestina, Alison H. Norris, Ann M. Moore, and Emily Freeman. 'Trajectories of Women's Abortion-Related Care: A Conceptual Framework'. *Social Science & Medicine* 200 (2018): 199–210.

Coast, Ernestina, Samantha R. Lattof, Yana van der Meulen Rodgers, Brittany Moore, and Cheri Poss. 'The Microeconomics of Abortion: A Scoping Review and Analysis of the Economic Consequences for Abortion Care-Seekers'. *PLoS One* 16, no. 6 (2021): e0252005.

Cohen, David S. and Carole Joffe. *Obstacle Course: The Everyday Struggle to Get an Abortion in America*. Oakland, California: University of California Press, 2020.

Collins, Patricia Hill. 'Black Women and Motherhood'. In *Motherhood and Space: Configurations of the Maternal through Politics, Home, and the Body*, edited by Sarah Hardy and Caroline Wiedmer, 149–59. New York: Palgrave Macmillan, 2005.

Conlon, Catherine. 'Concealed Pregnancy: A Case-Study Approach from an Irish Setting'. Crisis Pregnancy Agency, 2006. https://www.lenus.ie/bitstream/handle/10147/305217/approachformanIrishsetting.pdf (accessed 14 July 2023).

Connolly, Linda. 'The Women's Movement in Ireland, 1970–1995; A Social Movements Analysis'. *Irish Journal of Feminist Studies* 1, no. 1 (1996): 43–77.

Cornish, Flora, Jan Haaken, Liora Moskovitz, and Sharon Jackson. 'Rethinking Prefigurative Politics: Introduction to the Special Thematic Section'. *Journal of Social and Political Psychology* 4, no. 1 (2016): 114–27.

Corredor, Elizabeth S. 'On the Strategic Uses of Women's Rights: Backlash, Rights-Based Framing, and Anti-Gender Campaigns in Colombia's 2016 Peace Agreement'. *Latin American Politics and Society* 63, no. 3 (2021): 46–68.

Corwin, Julia E. and Vinay Gidwani. 'Repair Work as Care: On Maintaining the Planet in the Capitalocene'. *Antipode: A Radical Journal of Geography* (2021). Online First ahead of print 18 October 2021

Cox, Rosie. 'Some Problems and Possibilities of Caring'. *Ethics, Place and Environment* 13, no. 2 (2010): 113–30.

Daby, Mariela and Mason W. Moseley. 'Feminist Mobilization and the Abortion Debate in Latin America: Lessons from Argentina'. *Politics & Gender* 18, no. 2 (2022): 359–93.

Daigle, Megan, Deirdre N. Duffy, and Diana López Castañeda. 'Abortion Access and Colombia's Legacy of Civil War: Between Reproductive Violence and Reproductive Governance'. *International Affairs* 98, no. 4 (2022): 1423–48.

Danholt, Peter and Henriette Langstrup. 'Medication as Infrastructure: Decentring Self-Care'. *Culture Unbound* 4, no. 3 (2012): 513–32.

Darcy, Erin. *In Her Shoes: Women of the Eighth: A Memoir and an Anthology*. Ireland : New Island Books, 2020.

Darkwah, Akosua. 'Work as a Duty and as a Joy: Understanding the Role of Work in the Lives of Ghanaian Female Traders of Global Consumer Items'. In *Women's Labor in the Global Economy: Speaking in Multiple Voices*, edited by Sarah Hardy, 206–20. New Jersey: Rutgers University Press, 2007.

Darra, Susanne. '"Normal", "Natural", "Good" or "Good-Enough" Birth: Examining the Concepts'. *Nursing Inquiry* 16, no. 4 (2009): 297–305.

Davis, Angela Y. *Women, Race & Class*. New York: Vintage, 1983.

Davis, Jasmine Meredith, Casey Michelle Haining, and Louise Anne Keogh. 'A Narrative Literature Review of the Impact of Conscientious Objection by Health Professionals on Women's Access to Abortion Worldwide 2013–2021'. *Global Public Health* 17, no. 9 (2022): 2190–205.

de La Bellacasa, Maria Puig. *Matters of Care: Speculative Ethics in More Than Human Worlds*. Vol. 41. Minneapolis: University of Minnesota Press, 2017.

De Londras, Fiona and Mairead Enright. *Repealing the 8th*. Bristol: Policy Press, 2018.

De Londras, Fiona. '"A Hope Raised and Then Defeated"? The Continuing Harms of Irish Abortion Law'. *Feminist Review* 124, no. 1 (2020): 33–50.

de Souza, Natália Maria Félix and Lara Martim Rodrigues Selis. 'Gender Violence and Feminist Resistance in Latin America'. *International Feminist Journal of Politics* 24, no. 1 (2022): 5–15.

De Zordo, Sylvia, Giulia Zanini, Joanna Mishtal, Camille Garnsey, A.-K. Ziegler, and Caitlin Gerdts. 'Gestational Age Limits for Abortion and Cross-Border Reproductive Care in Europe: A Mixed-Methods Study'. *BJOG: An International Journal of Obstetrics & Gynaecology* 128, no. 5 (2021): 838–45.

Delay, Cara and Beth Sundstrom. '"In Her Shoes" and In Her Words: Voices, Silences, and Bodies in Irish Women's Abortion Narratives'. *Frontiers: A Journal of Women Studies* 43, no. 2 (2022): 139–68.

Deleuze, Gilles and Félix Guattari. *A Thousand Plateaus: Capitalism and Schizophrenia*. London: Bloomsbury Publishing, 1988.

Diedrich, Lisa. 'Que(e)rying the Clinic before AIDS: Practicing Self-Help and Transversality in the 1970s'. *Journal of Medical Humanities* 34 (2013): 123–38.

Drovetta, Raquel Irene. 'Safe Abortion Information Hotlines: An Effective Strategy for Increasing Women's Access to Safe Abortions in Latin America'. *Reproductive Health Matters* 23, no. 45 (2015): 47–57.

Drovetta, R. I. 'Stigma and Abortion in Argentina'. (2020; preprint). https://www.researchgate.net/profile/Raquel-Drovetta-2/publication/344692425_Stigma_and_Abortion_in_Argentina/links/5f89b71992851c14bccc40f2/Stigma-and-Abortion-in-Argentina.pdf (accessed 11 July 2023).

Duffy, Deirdre Niamh. 'From Feminist Anarchy to Decolonisation: Understanding Abortion Health Activism before and after the Repeal of the 8th Amendment'. *Feminist Review* 124, no. 1 (2020): 69–85.

Duffy, Deirdre Niamh, Claire Pierson, Caroline Myerscough, Diane Urquhart, and Lindsey Earner-Byrne. 'Abortion, Emotions, and Health Provision: Explaining Health Care Professionals' Willingness to Provide Abortion Care using Affect Theory'. *Women's Studies International Forum* 71 (2018): 12–18.

Duffy, Deirdre Niamh, Cordelia Freeman, and Sandra Rodríguez Castañeda. 'Beyond the State: Abortion Care Activism in Peru'. *Signs: Journal of Women in Culture and Society* 48, no. 3 (2023): 609–34.

Eagleton, Terry and Pierre Bourdieu. 'Doxa and Common Life'. *New Left Review* 191, no. 1 (1992): 115.

Eales, Lindsay and Danielle Peers. 'Care Haunts, Hurts, Heals: The Promiscuous Poetics of Queer Crip Mad Care'. *Journal of Lesbian Studies* 25, no. 3 (2021): 163–81.

Earner-Byrne, Lindsey and Diane Urquhart. *The Irish Abortion Journey, 1920–2018*. Basingstoke: Palgrave Macmillan, 2019.

Ellingson, Laura L. and Patricia J. Sotirin. 'Exploring Young Adults' Perspectives on Communication with Aunts'. *Journal of Social and Personal Relationships* 23, no. 3 (2006): 483–501.

Endler, Margit, Amanda Cleeve, Ingrid Sääv, and Kristina Gemzell-Danielsson. 'How Task-Sharing in Abortion Care became the Norm in Sweden: A Case Study of Historic and Current Determinants and Events'. *International Journal of Gynecology & Obstetrics* 150 (2020): 34–42.

Engle, Olivia. 'Abortion Mobilities'. *Geography Compass* 16, no. 9 (2022): e12656.

Engster, Daniel. 'Rethinking Care Theory: The Practice of Caring and the Obligation to Care'. *Hypatia* 20, no. 3 (2005): 50–74.

Enright, Mairead and Deirdre Duffy. 'Law and Childbirth in Ireland after the 8th Amendment: Notes on Women's Legal Consciousness'. *Journal of Law and Society* 49, no. 4 (2022): 753–77.

Epstein, Steven. 'Patient Groups and Health Movements'. In *The Handbook of Science and Technology Studies*, edited by Edward Hackett, Olga Amsterdamska, Michael Lynch, and Judy Wajcman, 499–541. Cambridge, MA: MIT Press, 2008.

Erdman, Joanna N. 'The Law of Stigma, Travel, and the Abortion-Free Island'. *Columbia Journal of Gender and Law* 33 (2016): 29.

Erdman, Joanna N., Kinga Jelinska, and Susan Yanow. 'Understandings of Self-Managed Abortion as Health Inequity, Harm Reduction and Social Change'. *Reproductive Health Matters* 26, no. 54 (2018): 13–19.

Ewig, Christina. 'Hijacking Global Feminism: Feminists, the Catholic Church, and the Family Planning Debacle in Peru'. *Feminist Studies* 32, no. 3 (2006): 633.

Feminist Critical Hindu Studies Collective. 'Auntylectuals: A Nonce Taxonomy of Aunty-Power'. *Text and Performance Quarterly* 42, no. 3 (2022): 346–57.

Ferreira, António and Enrica Papa. 'Re-Enacting the Mobility Versus Accessibility Debate: Moving Towards Collaborative Synergies Among Experts'. *Case Studies on Transport Policy* 8, no. 3 (2020): 1002–9.

Fitzsimons, Camilla. *Repealed: Ireland's Unfinished Fight for Reproductive Rights*. London: Pluto Press, 2021.

Fletcher, Ruth. 'Cheeky Witnessing'. *Feminist Review* 124, no. 1 (2020): 124–41.

Fletcher, Ruth. 'Negotiating Strangeness on the Abortion Trail'. In *Revaluing Care in Theory, Law and Policy: Cycles and Connections*, edited by Rosie Harding, Ruth Fletcher, and Chris Beasley, 14–30. London: Routledge, 2016.

Fletcher, Ruth. 'Silences: Irish Women and Abortion'. *Feminist Review* 50, no. 1 (1995): 44–66.

Foster, Diana Greene. *The Turnaway Study: Ten Years, a Thousand Women, and the Consequences of Having—Or Being Denied—An Abortion*. New York: Simon and Schuster, 2021.

Foucault, Michel. *Ethics: Subjectivity and Truth: Essential Works of Michel Foucault 1954–1984*. Penguin UK, 2019.

Foucault, Michel. *The Birth of the Clinic*. London: Routledge, 2012.

Freeman, Cordelia. 'Viapolitics and the Emancipatory Possibilities of Abortion Mobilities'. *Mobilities* 15, no. 6 (2020): 896–910.

Freeman, Cordelia and Sandra Rodríguez. 'The Chemical Geographies of Misoprostol: Spatializing Abortion Access from the Biochemical to the Global'. *Annals of the American Association of Geographers* 114, no. 4 (2024): 1–16.

Freire, Paulo. *Pedagogy of the Oppressed (Revised)*. New York: Continuum 356 (1996): 357–8.

Fricker, Miranda. *Epistemic Injustice: Power and the Ethics of Knowing*. Oxford: Oxford University Press, 2007.

Fried, Marlene Gerber. 'Reproductive Rights Activism in the Post-Roe Era'. *American Journal of Public Health* 103, no. 1 (2013): 10–14.

Furlong, Kathryn. 'Small Technologies, Big Change: Rethinking Infrastructure through STS and Geography'. *Progress in Human Geography* 35, no. 4 (2011): 460–82.

Furman, A. 'Desire Lines: Determining Pathways through the City'. *The Sustainable City VII: Urban Regeneration and Sustainability* 155 (2012): 23.

Ganchoff, Chris. 'Regenerating Movements: Embryonic Stem Cells and the Politics of Potentiality'. *Sociology of Health & Illness* 26, no. 6 (2004): 757–74.

Garnsey, Camille, Giulia Zanini, Silvia De Zordo, Joanna Mishtal, Alexandra Wollum, and Caitlin Gerdts. 'Cross-Country Abortion Travel to England and Wales: Results from a Cross-Sectional Survey Exploring People's Experiences Crossing Borders to Obtain Care'. *Reproductive Health* 18, no. 1 (2021): 1–13.

Gavigan, Shelley. 'The Criminal Sanction as it Relates to Human Reproduction: The Genesis of the Statutory Prohibition of Abortion'. *The Journal of Legal History* 5, no. 1 (1984): 20–43.

Gerdts, Caitlin, Silvia DeZordo, Joanna Mishtal, Jill Barr-Walker, and Patricia A. Lohr. 'Experiences of Women Who Travel to England for Abortions: An Exploratory Pilot Study'. *The European Journal of Contraception & Reproductive Health Care* 21, no. 5 (2016): 401–7.

Gill, Roopan K., Amanda Cleeve, and Antonella F. Lavelanet. 'Abortion Hotlines around the World: A Mixed-Methods Systematic and Descriptive Review'. *Sexual and Reproductive Health Matters* 29, no. 1 (2021): 75–89.

Gilmartin, Mary and Allen White. 'Interrogating Medical Tourism: Ireland, Abortion, and Mobility Rights'. *Signs: Journal of Women in Culture and Society* 36, no. 2 (2011): 275–80.

González-Vélez, Ana Cristina, Carolina Melo-Arévalo, and Juliana Martínez-Londoño. 'Eliminating Abortion from Criminal Law in Colombia: A Just Cause'. *Health and Human Rights* 21, no. 2 (2019): 85.

Gordon, Uri. 'Prefigurative Politics between Ethical Practice and Absent Promise'. *Political Studies* 66, no. 2 (2018): 521–37.

Gorman, Sally. 'Irish Actor Thanks British Hospitals for "Looking After Our Women in Their Time of Need" during BAFTA Speech'. *Irish Examiner*, 14 May 2018. https://www.irishexaminer.com/lifestyle/arid-30842740.html (accessed 10 July 2023).

Grabham, Emily. *Brewing Legal Times: Things, Form, and the Enactment of Law*. Toronto, Canada: University of Toronto Press, 2016.

Grimes, Lorraine, Joanna Mishtal, Karli Reeves, Dyuti Chakravarty, Bianca Stifani, Wendy Chavkin, Deirdre Duffy, et al. '"Still Travelling": Access to Abortion Post-12 Weeks Gestation in Ireland'. In *Women's Studies International Forum*, vol. 98, (2023): 102709.

Gustá, Ana Laura Rodriguéz. 'The Women's Movement in Argentina: Much Ado about Everything'. In *Twenty-First-Century Feminismos: Women's Movements in Latin America and the Caribbean*, edited by S. Bohn and C. Levy, 180–201. Canada: McGill-Queen's Press – MQUP, 2021.

Haaken, Jan. *Hard Knocks: Domestic Violence and the Psychology of Storytelling*. London: Routledge, 2010.

Habersang, Anja. 'Utopia, Future Imaginations and Prefigurative Politics in the Indigenous Women's Movement in Argentina'. *Social Movement Studies* Latest Issues (2022): 1–16DOI: 10.1080/14742837.2022.2047639.

Halfmann, Drew. 'Recognizing Medicalization and Demedicalization: Discourses, Practices, and Identities'. *Health* 16, no. 2 (2012): 186–207.

Hannam, Kevin, Mimi Sheller, and John Urry. 'Mobilities, Immobilities and Moorings'. *Mobilities* 1, no. 1 (2006): 1–22.

Hemmings, Clare. 'Resisting Popular Feminisms: Gender, Sexuality and the Lure of the Modern'. *Gender, Place & Culture* 25, no. 7 (2018): 963–77.

Hemmings, Clare. 'Telling Feminist Stories'. *Feminist Theory* 6, no. 2 (2005): 115–39.

Hemmings, Clare. *Why Stories Matter: The Political Grammar of Feminist Theory*. London: Duke University Press, 2011.

Hidayati, Isti, Wendy Tan, and Claudia Yamu. 'Conceptualizing Mobility Inequality: Mobility and Accessibility for the Marginalized'. *Journal of Planning Literature* 36, no. 4 (2021): 492–507.

Hillyard, Patrick A. R. *Suspect Community*. London: Pluto Press, 1992.

James, Stanlie Myrise and Abena P. A. Busia, eds. *Theorizing Black Feminisms: The Visionary Pragmatism of Black Women*. Psychology Press, 1993.

Jaramillo Sierra, Isabel C. 'The New Colombian Law on Abortion'. *International Journal of Gynecology & Obstetrics* 160, no. 1 (2023): 345–50.

Jeppesen, Sandra and Holly Nazar. 'Genders and Sexualities in Anarchist Movements'. In *The Continuum Companion to Anarchism*, edited by Ruth Kinna, 162–91. London, New York: Continuum International Publishing Group, 2012.

Joffe, Carole E., Tracy A. Weitz, and Clare L. Stacey. 'Uneasy Allies: Pro-choice Physicians, Feminist Health Activists and the Struggle for Abortion Rights'. *Sociology of Health &Illness* 26, no. 6 (2004): 775–96.

Kamal, Ohoud. 'Mundane Activism as a Mode of Urban Repair: A View from the Global South'. *Cities* 137 (2023): 104325.

Kaplan, Laura. *The Story of Jane: The Legendary Underground Feminist Abortion Service*. Chicago, IL: University of Chicago Press, 2019.

Khubchandani, Kareem. 'Between Aunties: Sexual Futures and Queer South Asian Aunty Porn'. *Porn Studies* 9, no. 3 (2022): 346–64.

Kidd, Ian James, José Medina, and Gaile Pohlhaus Jr, eds. *The Routledge Handbook of Epistemic Injustice*. Oxford, UK: Taylor & Francis, 2017.

Kim, Caron, Annik Sorhaindo, and Bela Ganatra. 'WHO Guidelines and the Role of the Physician in Task Sharing in Safe Abortion Care'. *Best Practice & Research Clinical Obstetrics & Gynaecology* 63 (2020): 56–66.

Kimport, Katrina. 'What to Know about the Costs of Traveling for Abortion Care in the US – Here's What I Learned from Talking to Hundreds of Women Who've Sought Abortions'. *The Conversation*, 30 August 2022. https://theconversation.com/what-to-know-about-the-costs-of-traveling-for-abortion-care-in-the-us-heres-what-i-learned-from-talking-to-hundreds-of-women-whove-sought-abortions-187266 (accessed 11 July 2023).

Kimport, Katrina, Tracy A. Weitz, and Lori Freedman. 'The Stratified Legitimacy of Abortions'. *Journal of Health and Social Behavior* 57, no. 4 (2016): 503–16.

Kittay, Eva Feder, and Ellen K. Feder, eds. *The Subject of Care: Feminist Perspectives on Dependency*. Oxford: Rowman & Littlefield, 2002.

Krajewska, Atina. 'Revisiting Polish Abortion Law: Doctors and Institutions in a Restrictive Regime'. *Social & Legal Studies* 31, no. 3 (2022): 409–38.

Larrea, Sara, Camila Hidalgo, Constanza Jacques-Aviñó, Carme Borrell, and Laia Palència. 'No One Should Be Alone in Living This Process'. *Sexual and Reproductive Health Matters* 29, no. 3 (2021): 213–25.

Latour, Bruno. *Reassembling the Social: An Introduction to Actor-Network-Theory*. Oxford: Oxford University Press, 2007.

Lawson, Victoria. 'Geographies of Care and Responsibility'. *Annals of the Association of American Geographers* 97, no. 1 (2007): 1–11.

Levesque, Jean-Frederic, Mark F. Harris, and Grant Russell. 'Patient-Centred Access to Health Care: Conceptualising Access at the Interface of Health Systems and Populations'. *International Journal for Equity in Health* 12 (2013): 1–9.

Lin, Cynthia S., Alisa A. Pykett, Constance Flanagan, and Karma R. Chávez. 'Engendering the Prefigurative: Feminist Praxes that Bridge a Politics of Prefigurement and Survival'. *Journal of Social and Political Psychology* 4, no. 1 (2016): 302–17

Lohr, Patricia A., Maria Lewandowska, Rebecca Meiksin, Natasha Salaria, Sharon Cameron, Rachel H. Scott, Jennifer Reiter, Melissa J. Palmer, Rebecca S. French, and Kaye Wellings. 'Should COVID-Specific Arrangements for Abortion Continue? The Views of Women Experiencing Abortion in Britain during the Pandemic'. *BMJ Sexual & Reproductive Health* 48, no. 4 (2022): 288–94.

Lord, Stephanie. 'The Logistics of Arranging Abortions'. *Feminist Ire: Not Your Fluffy Feminism*, 28 March 2013. https://feministire.com/2013/03/28/the-logistics-of-arranging-abortions/ (accessed 10 July 2023).

Lorde, Audre. *Sister Outsider: Essays and Speeches*. Berkeley, CA: Crossing Press, 2012.

Lowe, Pam and Sarah-Jane Page. *Anti-Abortion Activism in the UK: Ultra-Sacrificial Motherhood, Religion and Reproductive Rights in the Public Sphere*. Leeds, UK: Emerald Publishing Limited, 2022.

Luckert, Erika. 'Drawings We Have Lived: Mapping Desire Lines in Edmonton'. *Constellations* 4, no. 1 (2012): 318–27

Luna, Zakiya. *Reproductive Rights as Human Rights: Women of Color and the Fight for Reproductive Justice*. New York: NYU Press, 2020.

Macleod, Catriona Ida and John Hunter Reynolds. 'Reproductive Health Systems Analyses and the Reparative Reproductive Justice Approach: A

Case Study of Unsafe Abortion in Lesotho'. *Global Public Health* 17, no. 6 (2022): 801–14.

Macleod, Catriona Ida, Sian Beynon-Jones, and Merran Toerien. 'Articulating Reproductive Justice through Reparative Justice: Case Studies of Abortion in Great Britain and South Africa'. *Culture, Health & Sexuality* 19, no. 5 (2017): 601–15.

Macón, Cecilia, Mariela Solana, and Nayla Luz Vacarezza, eds. *Affect, Gender and Sexuality in Latin America*. Cham: Palgrave Macmillan, 2021.

Maffeo, Florencia, Natalia Santarelli, Paula Satta, and Ruth Zurbriggen. 'Parteras de nuevos feminismos: Socorristas en red—Feministas que abortamos;Una forma de activismo corporizado y sororo [Midwives of New Feminisms: Network of First Responders—Feminists who abort; A form of Embodied and Sisterly Activism]'. *Revista venezolana de estudios de la mujer [Venezuelan Journal of Women's Studies]* 20, no. 44 (2015): 217–27.

Mahon, Rianne and Fiona Robinson, eds. *Feminist Ethics and Social Policy: Towards a New Global Political Economy of Care*. Vancourver, BC, Canada: UBC Press, 2011.

Malvern, Chiwesh and Catriona Macleod. 'Cultural De-Colonization versus Liberal Approaches to Abortion in Africa: The Politics of Representation and Voice'. *African Journal of Reproductive Health* 22, no. 2 (2018): 49–59.

Margo, Judy, Lois McCloskey, Gouri Gupte, Melanie Zurek, Seema Bhakta, and Emily Feinberg. 'Women's Pathways to Abortion Care in South Carolina: A Qualitative Study of Obstacles and Supports'. *Perspectives on Sexual and Reproductive Health* 48, no. 4 (2016): 199–207.

Maroa, Janerose W. 'Assessing East Africa Community Initiatives in Managing Emerging Cross Border Criminal Trends'. PhD diss., University of Nairobi, 2013.

McGettrick, Claire, Katherine O'Donnell, Maeve O'Rourke, James M. Smith, and Mari Steed. *Ireland and the Magdalene Laundries: A Campaign for Justice*. London: Bloomsbury Publishing, 2021.

McLean, Robert, Grace Robinson, and James A. Densley. *County Lines: Criminal Networks and Evolving Drug Markets in Britain*. London: Springer Nature, 2019.

McQuinn, Cormac. 'Varadkar: 'It's Only a Matter of Time before a Woman Dies after Taking about Pills'. *Irish Independent*, 18 May 2018.

McReynolds-Pérez, Julia, Katrina Kimport, Chiara Bercu, Carolina Cisternas, Emily Wilkinson Salamea, Ruth Zurbriggen, and Heidi Moseson. 'Ethics of

Care Born in Intersectional Praxis: A Feminist Abortion Accompaniment Model'. *Signs: Journal of Women in Culture and Society* 49, no. 1 (2023): 63–87.

Mesman, Jessica. 'Resources of Strength: An Exnovation of Hidden Competences to Preserve Patient Safety'. In *A Socio-Cultural Perspective on Patient Safety*, edited by Emma Rowley and Justin Waring, 71–92. Aldershot, England: Ashgate, 2011.

Mignolo, Walter D. 'Introduction: Coloniality of Power and De-Colonial Thinking'. *Cultural Studies* 21, no. 2–3 (2007): 155–67.

Miremberg, Hadas, Oladayo Oduola, John J. Morrison, and Keelin O'Donoghue. 'Fetal Anomaly Diagnosis and Termination of Pregnancy in Ireland: A Service Evaluation Following Implementation of Abortion Services in 2019'. *American Journal of Obstetrics & Gynecology MFM* 5, no. 10 (2023): 101111.

Mishtal, Joanna, Karli Reeves, Dyuti Chakravarty, Lorraine Grimes, Bianca Stifani, Wendy Chavkin, Deirdre Duffy, et al. 'Abortion Policy Implementation in Ireland: Lessons from the Community Model of Care'. *Plos One* 17, no. 5 (2022): e0264494.

Mohamed, Fauzia and Mussa Ali Mussa. 'Emergence of Youth Criminal Groups Popularly Known as Panya Road and Ubaya Ubaya in Tanzania: The Case of Dar es Salaam City and Zanzibar Town'. *Research Journal of Education* 5, no. 7 (2019): 119–27.

Mol, Annemarie. *The Logic of Care: Health and the Problem of Patient Choice*. London: Routledge, 2008.

Moor, Robert. *On Trails: An Exploration*. New York: Simon and Schuster, 2016.

Morgan, Lynn M. 'The Dublin Declaration on Maternal Health Care and Anti-Abortion Activism: Examples from Latin America'. *Health and Human Rights* 19, no. 1 (2017): 41.

Morgan, Lynn M. and Elizabeth F. S. Roberts. 'Reproductive Governance in Latin America'. *Anthropology & Medicine* 19, no. 2 (2012): 241–54.

Motta, Sara C. 'Decolonising Critique: From Prophetic Negation to Prefigurative Affirmation'. In *Social Sciences for an Other Politics: Women Theorizing without Parachutes*, edited by Ana C. Dinerstein, 33–49. Cham, Switzerland: Springer Nature, 2017.

Motta, Sara C. *Liminal Subjects: Weaving (Our) Liberation*. New York: Rowman & Littlefield, 2018.

Moyle, Leah. 'Situating Vulnerability and Exploitation in Street-Level Drug Markets: Cuckooing, Commuting, and the "County Lines" Drug Supply Model'. *Journal of Drug Issues* 49, no. 4 (2019): 739–55.

Mullally, A., T. Horgan, M. Thompson, C. Conlon, B. Dempsey, and M. F. Higgins. 'Working in the Shadows, under the Spotlight–Reflections on Lessons Learnt in the Republic of Ireland after the First 18 Months of More Liberal Abortion Care'. *Contraception* 102, no. 5 (2020): 305–7.

Murphy Tighe, Sylvia and Joan G. Lalor. 'Concealed Pregnancy: A Concept Analysis'. *Journal of Advanced Nursing* 72, no. 1 (2016): 50–61.

Murphy, Michelle. 'Unsettling Care: Troubling Transnational Itineraries of Care in Feminist Health Practices'. *Social Studies of Science* 45, no. 5 (2015): 717–37.

Murray, Noëleen, Nick Shepherd, and Martin Hall, eds. *Desire Lines: Space, Memory and Identity in the Post-Apartheid City*. London: Routledge, 2007.

Nakanjako, Rita, Eria Olowo Onyango, and Robert Kabumbuli. 'Positioning Migrants in Informal Cross Border Trade: The Case of Busia, Uganda-Kenya Border'. *Eastern Africa Social Science Research Review* 37, no. 1 (2021): 123–43.

Nandagiri, Rishita. 'What's So Troubling about "Voluntary" Family Planning Anyway? A Feminist Perspective'. *Population Studies* 75 (2021): 221–34.

Nandagiri, Rishita and Lucía Berro Pizzarossa. 'Transgressing Biomedical and Legal Boundaries: The "Enticing and Hazardous" Challenges and Promises of a Self-Managed Abortion Multiverse'. In *Women's Studies International Forum*, vol. 100, 2023, 102799.

Nandagiri, Rishita, Ernestina Coast, and Joe Strong. 'COVID-19 and Abortion: Making Structural Violence Visible'. *International Perspectives on Sexual and Reproductive Health* 46 Supplement 1 (2020): 83–9.

Ngai, Mae M. *Impossible Subjects: Illegal Aliens and the Making of Modern America*. Princeton NJ: Princeton University Press, 2014.

Nyabola, Nanjala. 'Kenyan Feminisms in the Digital Age'. *Women's Studies Quarterly* 46, no. 3 & 4 (2018): 261–72.

O'Brien, Elizabeth and Miriam Rich. 'Obstetric Violence in Historical Perspective'. *The Lancet* 399, no. 10342 (2022): 2183–5.

O'Connor, Eva. *My Name is Saoirse*. London: Bloomsbury Publishing, 2015.

O'Donnell, Kelly Suzanne. 'Reproducing Jane: Abortion Stories and Women's Political Histories'. *Signs: Journal of Women in Culture and Society* 43, no. 1 (2017): 77–96.

O'donovan, Orla, Tiago Moreira, and Etaoine Howlett. 'Tracking Transformations in Health Movement Organisations: Alzheimer's Disease Organisations and their Changing "Cause Regimes"'. *Social Movement Studies* 12, no. 3 (2013): 316–34.

O'Malley, Evelyn. 'Taking the Ferry: Performing Queasy Affects through Irish Abortion Travel in Thorny Island and My Name is Saoirse'. *Contemporary Theatre Review* 29, no. 1 (2019): 23–38.

O'Shaughnessy, Aideen Catherine. 'Triumph and Concession? The Moral and Emotional Construction of Ireland's Campaign for Abortion Rights'. *European Journal of Women's Studies* 29, no. 2 (2022): 233–49.

O'Shea, Marie. *Independent Review on the Operation of the Health [Regulation of Termination of Pregnancy] Act 2018*. Department of Health/An Roinn Sláinte (Republic of Ireland), 2023. https://www.gov.ie/en/press-release/585fc-minister-for-health-publishes-the-review-of-the-operation-of-the-health-regulation-of-termination-of-pregnancy-act-2018-by-independent-chair-marie-oshea/ (accessed 19 February 2024).

Palmeiro, Cecilia. 'The Latin American Green Tide: Desire and Feminist Transversality'. *Journal of Latin American Cultural Studies* 27, no. 4 (2018): 561–4.

Paul, Mandira, Kristina Gemzell-Danielsson, Charles Kiggundu, Rebecka Namugenyi, and Marie Klingberg-Allvin. 'Barriers and Facilitators in the Provision of Post-Abortion Care at District Level in Central Uganda–A Qualitative Study Focusing on Task Sharing between Physicians and Midwives'. *BMC Health Services Research* 14 (2014): 1–12.

Pauw, Jacques. *Rat Roads: One Man's Incredible Journey*. Alexandria, Virginia: Zebra Press, 2012.

Petchesky, Rosalind P. *Abortion and Woman's Choice: The State, Sexuality, and Reproductive Freedom*. Boston, MA: Northeastern University Press, 1990.

Phipps, Alison. *Me, Not You: The Trouble with Mainstream Feminism*. Manchester, UK: Manchester University Press, 2020.

Pierson, Claire. *Prefigurative Politics of Care in Northern Ireland*. Conference presentation. University of Lincoln, 2023.

Pierson, Claire and Fiona Bloomer. 'Macro-and Micro-Political Vernaculizations of Rights: Human Rights and Abortion Discourses in Northern Ireland'. *Health and Human Rights* 19, no. 1 (2017): 173.

Pierson, C. and L. Caruana-Finkel. 'Abortion Care in Highly Restrictive Legal Regimes: The Experiences of Health and Social Care Professional in Malta'.

Briefing Paper, University of Liverpool, 2021. https://livrepository.liverpool.ac.uk/3128310/1/MaltaBriefingPaperMay2021FINAL.pdf (accessed 11 July 2023).

Pot, Mirjam. 'Epistemic Solidarity in Medicine and Healthcare'. *Medicine, Health Care and Philosophy* 25, no. 4 (2022): 681–92.

Power, Emma R. 'Assembling the Capacity to Care: Caring-with Precarious Housing'. *Transactions of the Institute of British Geographers* 44, no. 4 (2019): 763–77.

Power, Emma R. and Kathleen J. Mee. 'Housing: An Infrastructure of Care'. *Housing Studies* 35, no. 3 (2020): 484–505.

Power, Emma R., Ilan Wiesel, Emma Mitchell, and Kathleen J. Mee. 'Shadow Care Infrastructures: Sustaining Life in Post-Welfare Cities'. *Progress in Human Geography* 46, no. 5 (2022): 1165–84.

Power, Emma R., and Miriam J. Williams. 'Cities of Care: A Platform for Urban Geographical Care Research'. *Geography Compass* 14, no. 1 (2020): e12474.

Purnomo, Mangku, Ahmad Maryudi, Novil Dedy Andriatmoko, Edy Muhamad Jayadi, and Heiko Faust. 'The Cost of Leisure: The Political Ecology of the Commercialization of Indonesia's Protected Areas'. *Environmental Sociology* 8, no. 2 (2022): 121–33.

Qamar, Maria. *Trust No Aunty*. New York: Simon and Schuster, 2017.

Reagan, Leslie J. *When Abortion Was a Crime: Women, Medicine, and Law in the United States, 1867–1973, with a New Preface*. University of California Press, 2022.

Ribot, Jesse C. and Nancy Lee Peluso. 'A Theory of Access'. *Rural Sociology* 68, no. 2 (2003): 153–81.

Roberts, Celia, Imogen Tyler, Candice Satchwell, and Jo Armstrong. 'Health Social Movements and the Hybridisation of "Cause Regimes": An Ethnography of a British Childbirth Organisation'. *Social Movement Studies* 15, no. 4 (2016): 417–30.

Robinson, Fiona. 'Stop Talking and Listen: Discourse Ethics and Feminist Care Ethics in International Political Theory'. *Millennium* 39, no. 3 (2011): 845–60.

Rodgers, Dennis and Bruce O'neill. 'Infrastructural Violence: Introduction to the Special Issue'. *Ethnography* 13, no. 4 (2012): 401–12.

Romanis, Elizabeth Chloe and Jordan A. Parsons. 'Legal and Policy Responses to the Delivery of Abortion Care during COVID-19'. *International Journal of Gynecology & Obstetrics* 151, no. 3 (2020): 479–86.

Romanis, Elizabeth Chloe, Jordan A. Parsons, Isobel Salter, and Thomas Hampton. 'Safeguarding and Teleconsultation for Abortion'. *The Lancet* 398, no. 10299 (2021): 555–8.

Ross, Loretta J. 'African-American Women and Abortion: A Neglected History'. *Journal of Health Care for the Poor and Underserved* 3, no. 2 (1992): 274–84.

Rossiter, Anne. *Ireland's Hidden Diaspora – The 'Abortion Trail' and the Making of the London-Irish Underground, 1980–2000*. London: IASC Publishing, 2009.

Rosso, Laura. <<Alianzas estratégicas: Se lanzó Red Compañera, una organización para acompañar a personas que abortan>>. *Pagina 12*, 12 May 2021. https://www.pagina12.com.ar/343792-alianzas-estrategicas (accessed 10 July 2023).

Ruibal, Alba and Cora Fernandez Anderson. 'Legal Obstacles and Social Change: Strategies of the Abortion Rights Movement in Argentina'. *Politics, Groups, and Identities* 8, no. 4 (2020): 698–713.

Ruiter, Chelsea, Lance Hadley, and Queena Li. 'Impacts of Non-Tariff Barriers for Women Small Scale Cross-Border Traders on the Kenya-Uganda Border'. *Sauti Africa Journal* 2, no. 1 (2017): 1–9.

Salkever, David S. 'Accessibility and the Demand for Preventive Care'. *Social Science & Medicine (1967)* 10, no. 9–10 (1976): 469–75.

Segura-Ubiergo, Alex. *The Political Economy of the Welfare State in Latin America: Globalization, Democracy, and Development*. Cambridge: Cambridge University Press, 2007.

Sethna, Christabelle and Gayle Davis, eds. *Abortion across Borders: Transnational Travel and Access to Abortion Services*. Baltimore, MD: JHU Press, 2019.

Sethna, Christabelle and Marion Doull. 'Accidental Tourists: Canadian Women, Abortion Tourism, and Travel'. *Women's Studies* 41, no. 4 (2012): 457–75.

Shannon, Claude E. *Claude Elwood Shannon: Collected Papers*. New York : IEEE Press, 1993.

Sheldon, Sally, Gayle Davis, Jane O'Neill, and Clare Parker. *The Abortion Act 1967: A Biography of a UK Law*. Cambridge: Cambridge University Press, 2022.

Side, Katherine. '"A Hundred Little Violences, a Hundred Little Wounds": Personal Disclosure, Shame, and Privacy in Ireland's Abortion Access'. *Éire-Ireland* 56, no. 3 (2021): 181–205.

Side, Katherine. 'AB and C. versus Ireland: A New Beginning to Access Legal Abortion in the Republic of Ireland?'. *International Feminist Journal of Politics* 13, no. 3 (2011): 390–412.

Singer, Elyse Ona. 'Realizing Abortion Rights at the Margins of Legality in Mexico'. *Medical Anthropology* 38, no. 2 (2019): 167–81.

Skeggs, Beverley. *Becoming Respectable: Formations of Class and Gender*. New York: Sage, 1997.

Smith, Naomi and Peter Walters. 'Desire Lines and Defensive Architecture in Modern Urban Environments'. *Urban Studies* 55, no. 13 (2018): 2980–95.

Smyth, Lisa. *Abortion and Nation: The Politics of Reproduction in Contemporary Ireland*. Oxford: Routledge, 2017.

Spade, Dean. *Mutual Aid: Building Solidarity during this Crisis (And the Next)*. London: Verso Books, 2020.

Srinivasan, Sonia, Jessica R. Botfield, and Danielle Mazza. 'Utilising HealthPathways to Understand the Availability of Public Abortion in Australia'. *Australian Journal of Primary Health* 29, no. 3 (2022): 260–67

Stanley, Phiona. 'Unlikely Hikers? Activism, Instagram, and the Queer Mobilities of Fat Hikers, Women Hiking Alone, and Hikers of Colour'. *Mobilities* 15, no. 2 (2020): 241–56.

Stifani, Bianca M., Joanna Mishtal, Wendy Chavkin, Karli Reeves, Lorraine Grimes, Dyuti Chakravarty, Deirdre Duffy et al. 'Abortion Policy Implementation in Ireland: Successes and Challenges in the Establishment of Hospital-Based Services'. *SSM-Qualitative Research in Health* 2 (2022): 100090.

Stifani, Bianca M., Laura Gil Urbano, Ana Cristina Gonzalez Velez, and Cristina Villarreal Velasquez. 'Abortion as a Human Right: The Struggle to Implement the Abortion Law in Colombia'. *International Journal of Gynecology & Obstetrics* 143 (2018): 12–18.

Strebel, Ignaz, Alain Bovet, and Philippe Sormani. *Repair Work Ethnographies*. Singapore: Palgrave Macmillan, 2018.

Suh, Siri. 'Accounting for Abortion: Accomplishing Transnational Reproductive Governance through Post-Abortion Care in Senegal'. *Global Public Health* 13, no. 6 (2018): 662–79.

Sutton, Barbara. 'Reclaiming the Body: Abortion Rights Activism in Argentina'. *Feminist Formations* 33, no. 2 (2021): 25–51.

Sutton, Barbara and Nayla Luz Vacarezza, eds. *Abortion and Democracy: Contentious Body Politics in Argentina, Chile, and Uruguay*. Oxford: Routledge, 2021.

Swatuk, Larry A. and Peter Vale. '"A Better Life for All": Prefigurative and Strategic Politics in Southern Africa'. *Journal of Social and Political Psychology* 4, no. 1 (2016): 332–46.

Tamale, Sylvia. *Decolonization and Afro-Feminism*. Québec, Canada: Daraja Press, 2020.

Thomsen, Carly. 'The Politics of Narrative, Narrative as Politic: Rethinking Reproductive Justice Frameworks through the South Dakota Abortion Story'. *Feminist Formations* 7, no. 2 (2015): 1–26.

Thornton, James G. and Richard J. Lilford. 'Active Management of Labour: Current Knowledge and Research Issues'. *BMJ* 309, no. 6951 (1994): 366–9.

Tincknell, Estella. 'Monstrous Aunties: The Rabelaisian Older Asian Woman in British Cinema and Television Comedy'. *Feminist Media Studies* 20, no. 1 (2020): 135–50.

Tronto, Joan and Berenice Fisher. 'Toward a Feminist Theory of Caring'. In *Circles of Care*, edited by Emily K. Abel and Margaret Nelson, 29–42. Albany, NY: State University of New York Press, 1990.

Tronto, Joan C. *Moral Boundaries: A Political Argument for an Ethic of Care*. London: Psychology Press, 1993.

Tronto, Joan C. *Who Cares?: How to Reshape a Democratic Politics*. Ithaca, NY: Cornell University Press, 2015.

Truth, Justice, and Reconciliation Commission. 'Public Hearing Transcripts – Nyanza – Kisumu – RTJRC16.07 (H.H. The Aga Khan Hall, Kisumu) (Women's Hearing)'. I. Core TJRC Related Documents. 113, 2011. https://digitalcommons.law.seattleu.edu/tjrc-core/113 (accessed 11 July 2023).

Tsikata, Dzodzi. 'Gender, Land and Labour Relations and Livelihoods in Sub-Saharan Africa in the Era of Economic Liberalisation'. *Feminist Africa* 12 (2009): 11–30.

Tuck, Eve and K. Wayne Yang. 'Decolonization is not a Metaphor'. *Tabula Rasa* 38 (2021): 61–111.

Vacarezza, Nayla Luz and Julia Burton. 'Transformar los sentidos y el sentir. El activismo cultural de las redes de acompañantes de abortos en América Latina'. *Debate Feminista* 66 (2023): 1–30.

Vázquez, Rolando. 'Modernity Coloniality and Visibility: The Politics of Time'. *Sociological Research Online* 14, no. 4 (2009): 109–15.

Veldhuis, Suzanne, Georgina Sánchez-Ramírez, and Blair G. Darney. '"Becoming the Woman She Wishes You to Be": A Qualitative Study Exploring the Experiences of Medication Abortion Acompañantes in Three Regions in Mexico'. *Contraception* 106 (2022a): 39–44.

Veldhuis, Suzanne, Georgina Sánchez-Ramírez, and Blair G. Darney. 'Locating Autonomous Abortion Accompanied by Feminist Activists in the Spectrum of Self-Managed Medication Abortion'. *Studies in Family Planning* 53, no. 2 (2022b): 377–87.

Vivaldi, Lieta and Valentina Stutzin. 'Exploring Alternative Meanings of a Feminist and Safe Abortion in Chile'. In *Abortion and Democracy: Contentious Body Politics in Argentina, Chile, and Uruguay*, edited by Barbara Sutton and Nayla Luz Vacarezza, 226–45. Oxford: Routledge, 2021.

Walters, William. 'Migration, Vehicles, and Politics: Three Theses on Viapolitics'. *European Journal of Social Theory* 18, no. 4 (2015): 469–88.

Whitelaw, Sandy. 'Health Information: A Case of Saturation or 57 Channels and Nothing On?'. *The Journal of the Royal Society for the Promotion of Health* 128, no. 4 (2008): 175–80.

Wolfson, Mark. *The Fight Against Big Tobacco: The Movement, the State and the Public's Health*. Oxford: Routledge, 2017.

World Health Organization. *Towards a Supportive Law and Policy Environment for Quality Abortion Care: Evidence Brief*. Geneva: World Health Organization Human Reproductive Programme, 2022. https://www.who.int/publications/i/item/9789240062405 (accessed 31 January 2024).

World Health Organization. *Abortion Factsheet*. World Health Organization, 25 November 2021. https://www.who.int/news-room/fact-sheets/detail/abortion (accessed 30 January 2024).

Yates, Luke. 'Rethinking Prefiguration: Alternatives, Micropolitics and Goals in Social Movements'. *Social Movement Studies* 14, no. 1 (2015): 1–21.

Zordo, Silvia De. 'The Biomedicalisation of Illegal Abortion: The Double Life of Misoprostol in Brazil'. *História, Ciências, Saúde-Manguinhos* 23 (2016): 19–36.

Zurbriggen, Ruth, Brianna Keefe-Oates, and Caitlin Gerdts. 'Accompaniment of Second-Trimester Abortions: The Model of the Feminist Socorrista Network of Argentina'. *Contraception* 97, no. 2 (2018): 108–15.

Zurek, Melanie, Jenny O'Donnell, Rebecca Hart, and Deborah Rogow. 'Referral-Making in the Current Landscape of Abortion Access'. *Contraception* 91, no. 1 (2015): 1–5.

Index

abortion activism 17–18
  activist labour (burden of)
    55–6, 115
  differences between
    movements 117–19
  emotional labour 56
  experiences 57, 86–8, 97
abortion doulas 17, 157
abortion funds
  Abortion Support Network 17,
    161, 177
  National Network of Abortion
    Funds 17
abortion pathways 59
  sanctioned 135, 159
  surveillance 136
abortion pills 7, 10, 11, 121,
  156–7
  access to 16, 47
  misoprostol/mifepristone 9
  mobilities 40
  self-management 12, 135
abortion safety 12
abortion stigma 12, 17, 58, 85–6,
  137–8
abortion trail activism 179–84
abortion trail narratives
  as distinct from 130, 147
  legally outside 131–6
  lifelines 136–9, 162, 164
  risky 159, 172
  uncare 130
accessibility 41–2, 59
  dimensions of 43–4
  Peluso, Nancy Lee 37, 45
  Ribot, Jesse C. 37, 45
accompaniment 6–10, 29, 91–5,
  110, 143–4
  as a model of abortion care 17
  and prefiguration 110–12

Africa
  abortion activism 2, 10–12,
    84–5, 97–8
  abortion law 12–13
  abortion methods 85–6
  barriers to abortion access
    10–14, 113–14
  feminism 13–14
Ahmed, Sara 38, 60–3, 165, 170–1
Alam, Ashraful 18
alegal 135
anti-abortion legislation 154–5
Anzaldúa, Gloria 107–8
  counterstance 107, 118
Argentina
  abortion activism 6–7, 155
aunties/aunty 68–76
  African 54, 70, 74–6
  critical aunty studies 71
  cultural representations 69–71,
    73
  presence in abortion
    activism 54, 69
  role 4, 70
  satire 71
  South Asian 71–4
aunting schemas 70, 73–5

barriers to access
  cost 1, 13
  cultural 57–8
  epistemic 47–50, 53
  material 45–7, 113–14
  travel 143
Berro-Pizzarossa, Lucía 17, 42, 130,
  135, 157, 167
biomedical hegemony 118–19,
  159
Bloomer, Fiona 17, 131, 132, 153,
  155, 177

Index

Calkin, Sydney 16, 17, 40, 42, 93, 131, 132, 135, 156, 161
care
   abortion activism 84–5
   'crip' critiques 80
   feminist ethics 77–9, 83–4
   non-normative ontology 77, 80, 83–4
   supremacy 81
care collective 82
Center for Reproductive Rights 12, 154
Coast, Ernestina 16, 17, 38, 93
Colombia
   Corte Constitutionale 167–8
   legal changes 6, 31, 57–8, 155, 164–5
community health workers 119–20, 157
'constellation of actors' 17, 42
'county lines' 126, 179

decriminalization 6, 132, 155–8, 168
demedicalization 118, 157, 163
diversity work
   non-performative 60–2, 170
   phenomenological 38, 60, 62–4

Enright, Máiréad 4, 132, 160, 163, 176
epistemic privilege 48
epistemic solidarity 51, 54–5
Erdman, Joanna 7, 17, 130, 138
exnovation 141

Fletcher, Ruth 4, 5, 86, 177
Foucault, Michel 78, 79, 131, 133
Freeman, Cordelia 7, 9, 16, 17, 40, 42, 93, 116

health social movements 122, 162, 166, 172
   cause regimes 122, 172
   examples 122
   hybridization 165, 172

health systems and services
   activist collaborations with 117–19, 172
   inequality 8, 114, 136, 166–7
   privatisation 13
hermeneutic epistemic injustice 49–50
hot maps 9
Houston, Donna 18

information 9, 14, 158
   activism 50–1
   saturation 50
infrastructural turn 18
infrastructures 18, 89, 110, 164–6
   repair and maintenance 89–90, 93–4
   shadow 139–46
   unfinished 128
Ireland
   abortion law 3, 132, 160–3, 167, 170
   abortion travel 3–5, 86, 115, 167, 177
   availability of information 4–5
   ESCORT 51–2, 116, 161
   Irish Women's Abortion Support Group 4, 69, 161
   Liverpool Abortion Support Service (LASS) 1, 3–5, 38, 115–16, 161
   Liverpool Women's Hospital 176
   Society for the Protection of the Unborn Child (SPUC) 4
   Women's Information Network (WIN) 4, 161
Irish abortion services
   post-liberalisation 166–7

Jane
   Aunty Jane 54, 69–70
   Jane Collective 69–70

Kenya 12–13
Kirwan, Emmet 175, 176

Latin America
    abortion activism   6–10, 91–5, 118
    Marea Verde   6
    Ni Una Menos   6
    legality
        borders of   133–4
        knowledge   2, 96
Lord, Stephanie   31, 175, 177
Lorde, Audre   104

Maffeo, Florencia   6–7
MAMA Network   10, 38, 84
McReynolds-Pérez, Julia   18, 157
medical tourism   17, 179
mobility   39–41, 134
Moor, Robert   18–21, 24, 25, 27, 147, 179
Morgan, Lynn   8, 92, 167
mundane activism   145
mutual aid   104, 107

Nandagiri, Rishita   17, 42, 93, 130, 135, 157, 167
narrative politics
    abortion   11
    Hemmings, Claire   126–7
    modernity/decoloniality   126
Netherlands
    abortion access   14–16, 96
    migrants   96

'Old Left'   103, 105
O'Shea Review   167

panya
    cross-border trade   22–3
    cultural representations   21–2
    danger   21–2
    definition   21–5, 126, 128, 148
    gender   23
    history   23–4
    Pan-Africanism   24
    usage   22–5

Parceras   7, 57, 91
pharmacists   12, 119
Pierson, Claire   17, 101, 131, 153, 154, 177
Power, Emma   45, 90, 142–6
practical support
    activism   38
    logistics   47, 143
    networks   17
prefiguration
    contribution to analysis   121–2
    critiques   105–7
    definition   102–8
    presentism *vs.* future-building   105, 108
    reproductive justice   108–9, 123
pro-choice movement
    attitude to trails   151–3
    objectives   135, 146
Puig de la Bellacasa, Maria   77–9, 83, 90

'rat road'   21, 22, 179
Red Compañeras   1–2, 6, 16, 61, 95–8, 112, 118
reproductive governance   70, 83, 92, 112, 118, 167
reproductive justice   17, 81, 83, 102, 108, 122–3, 128–9, 147, 152–3, 156, 158–9, 165, 171, 182
Roberts, Elizabeth   8, 92, 167
Rossiter, Anne   4, 16, 69

Safe2Choose   54–5, 86
SisterSong Collective   123
Socorristas   2, 6–10, 38, 92–3, 95
Spade, Dean   104, 108

task-sharing   157
trails
    analytic value   125–6, 151–2, 179–80

colonialism 27
critical perspectives 26–8, 126–8
definitions 19, 126–7, 134
desire lines/*chemins de désir* 19–21, 126, 128
memory 27
political resistance 20
urban 19–21
Tronto, Joan C. 83–4, 89, 90

USA 94–5

Dobbs v Jackson Women's Health Centre 134, 136
Roe v Wade 134, 136
TRAP laws 136

Vacarezza, Nayla Luz 7, 17, 58, 91, 111, 163

World Health Organization 153–4, 157, 158

Zurbriggen, Ruth 91–3